Preface

C000010772

Enormous changes have taken place within British nursing over the past decade. New statutory bodies have been set up by the legislation resulting from the Report of the Committee on Nursing published in 1972. Implementation of Government policy has meant the closure and sale of the large hospitals for the mentally ill and handicapped; whilst there has been an enormous relative increase in the provision of private sector residential care for the increasing number of elderly people in our society. Widesweeping changes in the way the Health Service is managed were implemented in line with Griffiths' suggestion in the early part of the decade. A massive cultural change within the NHS followed the management changes. Yet it can be argued that the nursing care received by patients has developed enormously against the background of these changes.

These developments include the general acceptance of the Nursing Process, the introduction of nursing models, a recognition of the importance of holistic, individualized care and attention to the promotion and maintenance of quality of care. That these improvements in the provision of care have occurred says much for the adaptability and resilience of the nursing profession in the UK, because the decade has also seen the morale of nurses at a very low level indeed. Low morale occurred at the time of the implementation of the NHS management changes when the role of nurse managers was threatened. The implementation of the clinical grading structure in 1988, intended to reward those nurses who saw their career in clinical work, was interpreted by the bulk of the profession as threatening the status quo and morale plummeted again.

That the British nursing profession can develop and be strong in spite of much change presages well for the 1990s. The greatest change in Health Service provision in the UK since the inception of the NHS itself is beginning as I write. Changes in relation to the organization of community care will follow in about two years time. These will affect nursing in ways which are unpredictable.

In the meantime, a complete reorganization of nurse training, the so called Project 2000 reforms, are already underway. With these reforms, nurse training will be stronger academically, while still ensuring a broad practical experience during the course. However, the new type of nurse training foresees the need for trained nurses who engage in a broader role than has been the case in the past. Nurses trained in the Project 2000 programmes will understand more readily the health needs of the locality in which they work and the social pressures to which their clients and patients are subjected. They will be expected to have the knowledge and skills to engage in health promotion work, as well as the ability to care for those who are sick or disabled. Care will be focused more widely. In addition to hospitals, it will take place in people's family homes, residential homes and hostels to a greater extent than has occurred over the past 50 years or so. Nurses will rely more heavily on other carers, both informal (relatives, friends of the patients) and formal (health care assistants). The professional nurse may take on the leadership role in relation to the coordination of services to the client/patient

PRACTICAL NURSING

NURSES' AIDS SERIES

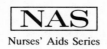

NAS

Nurses' Aids Series

PRACTICAL NURSING
HOSPITAL AND COMMUNITY NURSING
AND HEALTH PERSPECTIVES

Fourteenth Edition

Margaret Clarke

RGN, RNT, BSc (Hons), MPhil,
Orthopaedic Nursing Certificate (Hons),
Neurological and Neurosurgical Nursing Certificate
*Professor of Nursing Studies and Director of Institute of Nursing
Studies, University of Hull*; formerly *Ward Sister and Nurse Tutor, St
George's Hospital, London*

BAILLIERE TINDALL
London Philadelphia Toronto Sydney Tokyo

| Baillière Tindall | 24—28 Oval Road, |
| W.B. Saunders | London NW1 7DX |

The Curtis Center,
Independence Square West,
Philadelphia, PA 19106—3399, USA

55 Horner Avenue,
Toronto, Ontario M8Z 4X6, Canada

Harcourt Brace Jovanovich (Australia) Pty Ltd,
32—52 Smidmore Street,
Marrickville, NSW 2204, Australia

Harcourt Brace Jovanovich (Japan) Inc.
Ichibancho Central Building, 22-1 Ichibancho
Chiyoda-ku, Tokyo 102, Japan

© 1991 Baillière Tindall

All rights reserved. No part of this publication may be reproduced, stored in a retrieval system or transmitted, in any form or by any means, electronic, mechanical, photocopying or otherwise, without the prior permission of Baillière Tindall, 24—28 Oval Road, London NW1 7DX, UK.

First published 1938
Thirteenth edition 1983
Fourteenth edition 1991

Publisher's note
Miss Marjorie Houghton wrote the first nine editions of this book and the tenth in collaboration with Miss Mary Whittow.

Photoset by Setrite
Printed in Great Britain by Clays Ltd, St Ives plc

British Library Cataloguing in Publication Data

Clarke, Margaret
  Practical nursing—14th ed.—(Nurses' aids series)
  1. Practical nursing
  I. Title   II. Series
  610.73   RT62

ISBN 0-7020-1411-7

Contents

as keyworker, or may carry out a very circumscribed role in the assessment of nursing needs.

In all of this there is a danger that in taking on a new or changed role, the traditional role of the nurse will become eroded and devalued. This would be an enormous pity since the world wide reputation of the British nurse rests both on professionalism and practical ability.

In this latest edition of a book which has a long history of contributing to the practical knowledge of British nurses, the text has been expanded in the light of the imminent changes. However the traditional emphasis of the book has been safeguarded. Thus this edition includes health promotion perspectives in the chapters concerned with daily living activities and one chapter (Chapter 3) now includes a large new section devoted to health and individual behaviour. Community nursing perspectives are included whenever possible, but practical aspects of nursing interventions are still included within the later chapters of the book. In line with the trend in recent editions, the research basis for nursing practice has been identified and referenced and the importance of the psychosocial wellbeing of patients/clients is emphasized. Attempts to eliminate all gender bias led to language which was inelegant. Therefore, there are still many parts which refer to patients as he and nurses as she. The author recognizes and apologizes for any bias that this may imply. This language is used to aid clarity and avoid clumsiness.

It is difficult to include everything one would wish in a book which is as small as this one. I hope that this new edition serves to introduce the enquiring student nurse to the basics of nursing while whetting the appetite for seeking further information from other books and nursing journals.

Acknowledgements

My thanks to Sarah Smith, nursing editor at Baillière Tindall, for her enthusiasm and encouragement. Sandra Baulcomb, district nursing lecturer at Hull University helped enormously in ensuring that the community nursing perspective was realistic. Margaret McKeever and Susan Hamer, both academic staff in the Institute of Nursing Studies at Hull University, helped with their comments about current nursing practice.

Clearly other people have helped by discussing things with me and to these also, I say, thank you.

PART I: Introduction

1 The historical background of nursing

A study of the historical background of nursing is not only of great interest, it also enables us to understand and appreciate the influence of the past on professional nursing as we know it today. A few of the salient points are briefly outlined in this introductory chapter.

NURSING IN PAST AGES

Records of the early civilizations show that many of the diseases with which we are familiar are at least as old as history. Ancient India, Egypt, Assyria and Greece gave the physician a place of honour in civil life. Much of the practice of medicine was, however, inextricably mingled with religious practices. In the fourth century BC the Greek physician Hippocrates laid the foundation of rational medicine when he stated that disease was due to disordered function of the body, often the result of disobeying the laws of health, and not to the work of evil spirits or the wrath of the gods, as was formerly believed. His treatment was based on close clinical observation of symptoms and signs, and his medical notes, clearly but simply written, are still regarded as models.

However, even in Hippocrates' time we find no mention of skilled nursing by specially trained attendants. Treatment was carried out by the physician or his pupil assistants, and the general nursing care of the patient was in the hands of the women of the household or of slaves. It is worth noting that a large proportion of the nursing care of the sick has continued to be carried out by women of the household throughout history. This is as true today as it ever was. Midwives are frequently mentioned in early days, and midwifery was usually a hereditary family profession. The 'man midwife' and the obstetric physician were innovations of the seventeenth century.

THE CHRISTIAN ERA

The teachings of Christ that service to the very humblest living creature was service to God, and that it was the duty and privilege of the strong to bear the burdens of the weak, inspired the early Christians to seek out those needing help, and to go beyond the narrow limits of their own homes ministering to the bodily and spiritual needs of the sick and poor. The Order of Deaconesses was formed and, working with the Deacons under the Bishops, became the first organized visiting service. A group of wealthy and influential Roman matrons, friends and followers of St Jerome in the fourth century AD, also included nursing among their Christian duties, although they did not form an order.

In the medieval period, when the Church was the great intellectual and social force in all the countries of Christendom, the religious orders were responsible for the care of all who needed help, whether from sickness, poverty or old age. It is interesting to note that many of the large monasteries (some housed 3000 inmates) had houses both for monks and for nuns, and that the supreme control of the dual establishment was often in the hands of a woman, the Abbess. The Abbesses were undoubtedly great figures in their day and age. Their knowledge was wide and their administrative abilities of a very high order.

At the time of the Crusades, in the twelfth century, the military orders were founded. The most powerful and the most famous was the Order of the Knights Hospitallers of St John of Jerusalem. This order had a 'langue' or branch in every country of Christendom. They founded and maintained hospitals, first in Jerusalem and later in Rhodes and Malta. The nursing was performed by 'serving brothers', but there was a subsidiary women's order whose members nursed in the hospital at Jerusalem, though not in any other hospital of the Order. In the sixteenth century the Order was suppressed in this country, but was re-established in a different form in the nineteenth century. Now everyone is familiar with at least some of its activities, the St John Ambulance Association and the Voluntary Nursing Corps being the best known.

The Sisters of Charity

In France in the seventeenth century the most important nursing order was that of the Augustinian Sisters. They staffed the largest Paris hospital, the Hôtel-Dieu. These sisters must have been very overworked. The practice, common at that time, of putting as many as six patients in one bed, made their wards very overcrowded, and in addition to nursing they had to do domestic work, including the washing, which they did in the Seine. Their nursing work was also necessarily limited by the required attention to religious duties, their working day being directed by the priests and not by the physicians. It was not considered suitable that celibate nuns should know much about their patient's bodies or their diseases, so that efficient nursing was hardly possible. The sisters led a life of total self-abnegation and gave loyal and kindly service to the sick, but in those circumstances it was quite impossible that the sick could receive adequate nursing care.

A French priest, Vincent de Paul (afterwards canon-ized), took an extremely practical interest in the adminis-tration of charity, both in hospitals and in the homes of the poor, and when visiting the Hôtel-Dieu he was greatly impressed by the need for a more efficient service. With the aid of several influential ladies who had worked with him under the name of 'Dames de Charité' in a voluntary visiting service, he took a house in Paris, and there gath-ered a group of country girls of good character who were to be trained to work in the Hôtel-Dieu with the Augustinian Sisters. His great helper was a Mlle Le Gras, who became the first Superior of the Sisters of Charity, the nursing community which grew from this small beginning.

St Vincent instructed the sisters that they were to give implicit obedience to the physicians (this was very revol-utionary teaching) and that they must take no vows nor be tied to a cloistered life, but go wherever they were needed. Indeed, it was not long before the sisters were to be found all over the country, nursing in the homes of the people, in hospitals and in homes for the aged and insane, and from 1654 they rendered service on the battle-field in many campaigns. It is noteworthy that St Vincent considered that their general as well as their professional education was important, and wished the sisters to have instruction in reading, writing and arithmetic.

The Dark Ages of English nursing

From the disestablishment of the monastic orders by Henry VIII until the reforms of the nineteenth century, England had no nursing orders comparable with the Augustinian Sisters or the Sisters of Charity. The existing charitable foundations had to staff their institutions with such women as they were able to hire, and the status of nurses was hardly as good as that of a domestic servant in a good-class house. In the wealthier private house the patient was nursed by the women of the household or by 'professional' nurses. 'Handywomen' were available to care for the sick of the poor who had no relatives to care for them (Dingwall et al, 1988). Charles Dickens has left us a caricature of the handywoman in his description of Sairey Gamp. The public conscience awakened slowly, stirred by the pioneers and progressive leaders in all branches of science and the professions. The more advanced physicians advocated the training of educated women for real nursing service; the religious bodies, especially the Society of Friends, felt that the appalling social conditions so largely due to ignorance and neglect must be remedied. The latter half of the nineteenth century also saw great advances in medicine, surgery and all scientific knowledge.

Nursing reforms of the pre-Nightingale period

The examples of the communities of the Sisters of Charity in France and the Deaconess Institute at Kaiserswerth near Düsseldorf in Germany inspired the foundation of the many communities in this country in the middle of the nineteenth century. The Kaiserswerth Institute was a new venture that was fast proving itself eminently successful. A German pastor and his wife, Theodore and Frederica Fliedner, had started a small home for discharged women prisoners, and had shortly afterwards added a hospital to their activities. Here they trained a succession of young women of good character and upbringing to be deaconesses. Their duties included nursing in hospital and in the home, home management and the care of young children, and religious visiting. They received practical instruction from the pastor's wife, theoretical instruction in their professional duties from the physicians, and ethical lectures from the pastor. It was an attempt to give an organized training; and though Florence Nightingale, who received practical hospital training at the Institute, clearly saw that the nursing and hygiene could be improved, she was greatly impressed by the moral tone.

Mrs Elizabeth Fry, of the Society of Friends, knew the Fliedners and their work, and one of her many activities was to found the Protestant Nursing Sisters in 1840. The Park Village Community in north-west London was the first order under the Church of England, but the work of its members was that of visiting rather than nursing. Miss Sellon in Devonport was the head of a band of Sisters of Mercy who gained most of their nursing experience in all too frequent epidemics. Some of these sisters accompanied Miss Nightingale to the Crimea and were often referred to by her as the 'Sellonites'.

In 1845 St John's House was started as a training school for nurses under religious direction. The head of the community was a priest of the Anglican Church. The nurses went to King's College Hospital for practical experience and also received instruction from the doctors at the hospital. Later this order took over the entire nursing in that hospital until a lay training school was established in 1885. The St John Sisters also nursed in the Metropolitan and Charing Cross Hospitals.

The sisters of another Church community, that of All Saints, nursed in the wards of University College Hospital for more than 20 years.

THE NIGHTINGALE ERA

When Miss Nightingale was asked by the Secretary at War, Sidney Herbert, to take a band of nurses out to the Crimea to give the same care to our soldiers that the Sisters of Charity were already giving to the French, the great opportunities of a life of preparation for such a task had come.

This woman of wide education and high social position had from her youth been imbued with the idea that the care and comfort of the sick, and the promotion of health in the family, was work for women of character and education. In spite of home opposition she managed to see all that there was to see of training on the Continent; she was, however, to set standards of practical nursing and hospital administration far in advance of any that she found. At the time of the Crimean War Miss Nightingale was in charge of a small hospital for gentlewomen in Chandos Street.

Her first difficulty when she accepted the task of organizing a nursing service for the army in the Crimea was to find a sufficient number of experienced nurses of reliable character, and to refuse the numerous offers from the totally untrained and unfitted. Florence Nightingale saw that in many quarters this innovation of women in the army hospitals would not meet with favour, and she was most anxious not to take the type of woman who would make the work yet more difficult.

When she arrived in Scutari she found a lack of all provision for the care and comfort of the sick and wounded, and an indifference to this dreadful state of affairs that aroused her to a fury of organization and unsparing work. Conditions were as difficult as they could possibly be, red tape obstructed her on all sides, the army doctors resented the presence of women and, sad to record, her nurses did not all prove suitable, some drank, some were unable to stand the dreadful conditions, others found her a hard supervisor and were continually bickering. Certainly Miss Nightingale spared none, herself least of any.

The soldiers looked upon her as an angel, officialdom regarded her in quite another light, but the public made her their national heroine, and when she returned, broken in health, a grateful country presented her with a large sum of money (£9000 of which had been subscribed by private soldiers). With this money she founded the Nightingale Training School at St Thomas's Hospital. The pupils in this school were 'trained to train', so that they could in their turn fill important nursing posts throughout the country; and this was only one of the activities of a woman who was almost a continual invalid for the rest of her life, but it was one to which she gave much personal attention.

In addition to laying the firm foundations of the modern system of nursing training, this one woman was responsible for the complete reorganization of civil and military hospitals, and for many reforms improving the sanitation and hygiene of the army, particularly in India.

Much emphasis has been placed on the role of Florence Nightingale in shaping the nursing profession as we know it today. However, no nurse who is interested in his or her profession can afford to ignore other historical strands which contribute in terms of influence if not in terms of image to nursing as we know it. Two of the other roots come from the Poor Law Nursing Service (White, 1978) and the Asylums (Carpenter, 1980). A knowledge of Poor Law Nursing challenges us to think of 'care' rather than 'cure'. A history of Asylum nursing challenges us to think about the custodial role of the nurse and the effects of institutionalization, not only on patients but also on staff. Carpenter (1980) also claims that from 'Asylum nurses' comes the pressure toward trade unionism in nursing. The remaining influence on nursing comes from the community, both from the Nightingale-influenced district nurses and health visitors whose origin appears to stem from the Ladies Sanitary Reform Association in Manchester and Salford from 1862 (Owen, 1977).

PROFESSIONAL ORGANIZATION

The increasing demand for the 'Nightingale Nurses' and the opening up of this new profession to educated women meant, of course, that the profession increased rapidly in numbers, and the question of organization and registration on the lines already instituted for the medical profession soon arose. Miss Nightingale herself was opposed to state registration. She always regarded nursing as a vocation, not as a profession, but it is strange that this far-sighted woman could not see the necessity for protecting both the public and the nurses from exploitation by those who were untrained or partly trained.

There is no doubt that the opposition of the most influential person in the nursing world must have been a great factor in delaying state registration for so many years.

The first organized body of trained nurses was that formed by Mrs Bedford Fenwick in 1887 and known as the British Nurses' Association. Mrs Bedford Fenwick, before she married Dr Bedford Fenwick, was Miss Gordan Manson, Matron of St Bartholomew's Hospital. The British Nurses' Association was incorporated by Royal Charter and became the Royal British Nurses' Association. With much opposition from within the profession and from without, efforts were made to get a Nurses' Registration Bill through Parliament, but without success. The first Registration Act was passed in 1901, not in England, but in New Zealand.

In 1894 the Matrons' Council of Great Britain and Ireland was formed. In 1898 the Council wholeheartedly accepted Mrs Bedford Fenwick's proposals for an International Council of Nurses. The object was to admit to membership all national nursing groups which had developed, or were trying to develop, professional self-government and a settled professional status. The International Council is mainly concerned with organizing international interchange of nurses, promoting the advance of nursing service and nursing education and the economic and social welfare of nurses throughout the world. It has links with a number of international organizations, including the World Health Organization.

During the long period from 1887 until after the First World War the struggle for registration in England dragged on. In 1916 the College of Nursing was founded by leaders of the nursing profession and by other influential persons impressed with the need for greater professional organization. A draft scheme for the State Registration Act was drawn up. With amendments to this and to the original Bill presented by the Royal British Nurses' Association, a New Bill was sponsored by the Minister of Health, and became, in 1919, the Nurses' Registration Act.

The College of Nursing was granted a Royal Charter in 1929; it is now the Royal College of Nursing with headquarters in Cavendish Square, London, and branches throughout England and Wales. A Scottish Board in Edinburgh and a Northern Ireland Committee in Belfast are local headquarters for the Scottish and Northern Ireland Branches. It is the largest organization of registered nurses in the UK and its activities are many. The professional association department of the College is chiefly concerned with forming and implementing professional policies and giving help where required to the individual nurse. The educational side of the activities of the College covers a wide field in preparing nurses for posts in hospitals and in the fields of public health and occupational health, including preparation for teaching and administration in all these areas.

The United Kingdom organization in membership with the International Council of Nurses was the National Council of Nurses of Great Britain and Northern Ireland, a federation of professional associations, nurses' leagues and fellowships. In 1962 agreement was reached between the National Council and the Royal College of Nursing that the two bodies should amalgamate to form one united organization which would in future represent British nursing internationally under the name of the 'Royal College of Nursing and National Council of Nurses of the United Kingdom'. Membership of the new organization is on an individual basis and this national body is therefore no longer a federation of associations and leagues and it should be noted that all registered and enrolled nurses, whether on the general or another part of the Registers maintained by the United Kingdom Central Council (UKCC) are eligible to apply for membership of the Royal College of Nursing and National Council of Nurses.

THE STATE AND NURSING

As has already been stated, the first Nurses' Registration Act was placed on the Statute Book in 1919. This Act established the General Nursing Council for England and Wales as the statutory body responsible for forming and maintaining the Register of Nurses. Similar Acts established Nursing Councils with the same functions in Scotland and Ireland. The Council also had the duty of laying down conditions for the approval of hospitals as training schools for nurses, inspection of conduct of hospitals so approved, and examinations for admission to the Register. Separate parts of the Register were set up for general trained nurses and for nurses trained in the care of sick children, fever patients and patients suffering from mental illness and mental deficiency. Originally there was a separate part of the Register for general trained male nurses, but this part was subsequently amalgamated with the part of the Register for general trained female nurses.

No further nursing legislation was enacted until 1943, when, under the Nurses Act, 1943, the Council was charged with the duty of forming and maintaining a Roll of Assistant Nurses, inspecting and approving hospitals where such training could be undertaken, and conducting examinations for admission to the Roll. The type of examination which the Council considered appropriate for this type of training was mainly concerned with the candidates' practical nursing ability and was known as the 'assessment'. Under the 1943 Act the right to use the title of 'nurse' was, with a few exceptions approved by the Minister of Health, limited to registered nurses, en-rolled assistant nurses and students or pupil nurses under-going training for admission to the Register or Roll. This Act also gave the Council the responsibility of registering as registered nurse tutors those nurses who are qualified in teaching in schools of nursing.

In 1949 further nursing legislation was enacted, and this Act was designed primarily to 'improve the training of nurses for the sick'. The main provisions of the Act as it affected nurse training were to give further powers to the General Nursing Council, to enlarge the representation on the Council, and to set up in each of the regional hospital areas, Area Nurse Training Committees con-cerned with regional matters relating to the training of nurses. From 1 April 1974, following the National Health Service Reorganisation Act (1972), these became Regional Nurse Training Committees. One provision implemented, at least partially, a recommendation of both the Athlone and the Horder Committees, namely that finance required for the education and training of nurses should be separated from the expenditure required for the maintenance of the hospital services. In 1957 a further Act consolidated the previous three Nursing Acts of 1919, 1943 and 1949. A private member's Bill, introduced into Parliament by Dame Irene Ward in 1960, had as its main objective the removal of the word 'assistant' from the title of the enrolled nurse. This Bill was supported by both parties in the House of Commons and was entered on the Statute Book in March 1961. It is a measure of the value of the work of the enrolled nurse and the recognition of her place in the nursing profession that this measure had the wholehearted support of the majority of registered nurses.

A fairly recent development in nurse training was the setting up of integrated and experimental courses of nurse education. One type of course was the integrated course in which general nurse training, community nurse training, and health visitor training were combined in a four-year course. A course of this kind at Manchester University was the first course in England, on the successful completion of which the student is awarded a degree in nursing. A degree course with nursing as the major subject has been offered at Edinburgh University for some years.

Several universities and polytechnics now offer courses in which an honours degree may be combined with nurse training, whilst several hospitals offer a two-year nurse training course leading to state registration for university graduates.

It should be noted that the duties and responsibilities of the nursing statutory bodies are clearly defined and limited by Act of Parliament and by Statutory Rules approved by the Minister of Health.

In 1970, the Joint Board of Clinical Studies was set up. This controlled the training and examination of all students of post-basic training not the concern of the General Nursing Council, the Central Midwives Board or the Council for the Education and Training of Health Visitors. Following the Report of the Briggs' Committee on Nursing, published in 1972 (Cmnd 5115), new statutory bodies were made responsible for nurse education and training and for keeping a Register of nurses, midwives and health visitors by 1 September 1983 at the latest. These new bodies comprise the UK Central Council and National Boards for England, Wales, Scotland and Northern Ireland. For the first time, nurses are all overseen by the same bodies. There is provision in the Nurses, Midwives and Health Visitors Act (1979) for a single professional register.

Whilst the structural recommendations of the Briggs' Committee were eventually implemented, the educational recommendations were put to one side (Dingwall et al, 1988). However, the Royal College of Nursing continued to press for educational reforms, culminating in the publication of a report from a committee set up by the Royal College of Nursing (Royal College of Nursing, 1985). Publication of this report coincided with fears about future recruitment to the nursing profession in the face of the projected shortage of 18-year-old females in the first half of the 1990s. Two other reports followed in quick succession: one from the English National Board (1985), the other from the UKCC (1986). The UKCC Project 2000 report is currently being implemented (1989—1993), although some bargaining with the health departments has resulted in changes from the original document. Nurse training of the future will embody the following features:

1. Trainees will have student status. They will be supported by a non-means-tested bursary rather than a salary, but they will be regarded as contributing 20% of their time to service.

2. An 18-month common foundation programme will be followed by an 18-month 'branch programme' leading to registration on the general, paediatric, mental health or mental handicap parts of the Register. Direct entry into midwifery training is to be encouraged.

3. During the course, students will be educated to act as health promoters as well as caring for the sick. They will be prepared for work in the community as well as in hospitals.

4. Links of various kinds are to be forged with higher/ further education and the qualification gained is to have academic validity as well as professional recognition.

A separate trend, favoured by regional health authorities and taken up by health educational bodies, is for the amalgamation of separate Schools of Nursing into Colleges where nurse education is not completely absorbed into higher education.

A further working paper annexe to the Government's recent White Paper on the Health Service has been published (DHSS, 1989b), (see later for further details) and includes the following features:

1. Regional health authorities will have a major role in planning training to ensure adequate staff for each region. They will bear the costs of preregistration training and, in the case of midwifery, they will bear the costs for both direct entry and postregistration courses.

2. The role of the statutory nurse training bodies is reviewed.

3. Regional funding is envisaged for health visiting, district nursing, community psychiatric nursing and community mental handicap nursing courses.

4. Contracts would be negotiated between health auth-

orities and training institutions to cover:
(a) Allocation of funds to training institutions
(b) Number of students to be trained
(c) Student support
(d) Cost of student placements
(e) Teaching and supervision in the workplace during placements
(f) A statement of training outcomes
(g) A statement of how contract compliance is to be monitored.

The implementation of the National Health Service Act on 5 July 1948, brought all hospitals, with a few exceptions, under State ownership. Under this Act every man, woman and child in the country is entitled to medical attention and hospital treatment as and when required. Medical and nursing treatment is available without charge to the individual. The full cost of the National Health Service, paid for by taxation, represents a very considerable proportion of the total national income, but few argue against its importance for the nation and the individual. This financial burden, long accepted as right and necessary both as a means of alleviating suffering and promoting a standard of health vital for the future well-being of the nation, is currently questioned. Alternative ways of financing the Health Service are frequently under discussion. It follows then that it is the duty of all who participate in this work not only to endeavour to foster and maintain high standards of service but also to accept responsibility for ensuring that the nation's money is expended to the best advantage.

On the inauguration of the National Health Service hospitals, general practitioner services and local health services were administered separately from one another.

In a report on the National Health Service (Green

Paper: *The Future Structure of the National Health Service*, 1970) it was proposed that area health authorities should administer hospital and specialist services, family practitioner, ambulance, community health and nursing services, family planning clinics and the school health service, thus unifying the three separate aspects of the National Health Service.

A Bill based on these proposals was passed in 1972 and implemented on 1 April 1974 following consultation with the professions involved. Services brought together under the same authorities were:

1. Hospital and specialist services
2. Family practitioner services
3. Personal health services, formerly administered by local health authorities
4. The school health service, previously administered by the local education authority.

Personal health services include ambulance services, family planning, health centres, health visiting, home nursing, maternity and child health. Thus preventive and curative services were brought together under the same authority.

There were three levels of health authority: regional, area and district health authorities. The smallest of these were the districts which are responsible for the health service provision of populations ranging from 150 000 to 300 000 people. Area health authorities administered between one and six districts. There are 14 regional health authorities, each with one or more university medical schools within its boundaries.

From 1 April 1982, area health authorities disappeared and the administration of the health services rested with the regional health authorities, family practitioner comitees and newly appointed district health authorities.

The latter were appointed by the Secretary of State and represent local authorities, the universities, etc.

Acceptance by the Government of the recommendations outlined by Sir Roy Griffiths in 1984 brought about a change in the way that the National Health Services were managed. District general managers were appointed to head up each health district. They were responsible for the organization's performance in delivering health services to the population of the district. Decision making, including the holding of budgets, was to be devolved to the lowest level possible within the organization. These changes were implemented over a period of time to a varying degree within different health authorities. Where they were successfully implemented it meant, for example, that ward sisters and charge nurses became budget holders for the first time, allowing them to make judgements about priorities for funding within the ward.

The Government's White Paper, *Working for Patients* (DHSS, 1989a), introduces an element of competitiveness into the provision of health care. Hospitals and community services become contractors, offering their services at a stated price. District health authorities and/or general practitioners will have a budget to buy services, other than core services, at the best price they can obtain. Some hospitals will become self-governing trusts. District health authorities will become smaller, consisting of five executive and five non-executive members.

Following the successful application by the United Kingdom to join the European Economic Community, nursing directives were signed in 1977. The first of these directives is concerned with the mutual recognition of diplomas and facilitation of freedom of individual nurses to provide nursing service within the member states. Basically, in the case of British nurses, in order to practise in the European Community, they must:

1. Hold a registered nurse qualification (1st level).
2. Have practised recently in the UK.
3. Have the linguistic knowledge necessary for practice.

However, the second directive is more important in many ways as it is concerned with the programme of training for registration. Requirements are:

1. Ten years of general education as a minimum requirement before entry to nurse training.
2. Adequate knowledge of the sciences on which nursing is based; sufficient knowledge of the nature and ethics of the professions and of the general principles of health and nursing; adequate clinical experience under the supervision of qualified staff; ability to participate in the training of health personnel; experience of working with other professions in the health sector.
3. Clinical instruction must be undertaken in medicine, surgery, child care and paediatrics, maternity care, mental health and psychiatry, care of the old and geriatrics and home nursing (Quinn, 1980).

In practice, this second directive has meant a reorganization of nurse training for the register to ensure that all student nurses gain the necessary experience.

MENTAL HEALTH

The treatment and care of persons suffering from mental illness or mental handicap even at the beginning of the century was largely limited to custodial care which had as its object preventing the patient from harming himself or other people. The admission of patients and the administration of mental institutions were largely dictated by Acts of Parliament: the Lunacy and Mental Treatment Acts of 1890 to 1930 and the Mental Deficiency Acts of 1913 to 1938. Towards the end of the nineteenth century the Royal Medico-Psychological Association, a professional association of doctors primarily concerned with, and interested in, the treatment of mental illness and mental deficiency, initiated a course of training and an examination for men and women working in mental hospitals and mental deficiency hospitals and at that time referred to as 'attendants'. This step marks the beginning of true professional nursing in these fields. Since then great advances have been made not only in the medical treatment but also in the nursing care of the mentally disordered. As interest in and knowledge of mental illness increased, so the old conditions in the asylums, with their padded cells, strait-jackets and locked doors, gave way to the development of the mental hospital as a 'therapeutic community'. The psychological, physical and social methods used in the treatment of mental patients now make this a field of service for the nurse where therapeutic planning, intelligent understanding, sympathy and an ability to form good personal relationships are of outstanding importance.

The Mental Health Act, 1959, which has been implemented in stages since October 1959, provides for the treatment of patients suffering from mental disorders on the same basis as that of patients suffering from any type of physical illness. Admission to hospital in the case of mental illness or mental subnormality is now 'informal'; that is to say the legal requirement that the patient should first be certified as being 'of unsound mind' no longer operates, although there is provision for compulsory detention in certain circumstances where this is in the interests of the patient and the public. The Act also places responsibilities on health authorities to provide for the care of the mentally sick and subnormal in the community.

Current policy (1989–1993) is aimed at the closure of

large institutional hospitals for mentally ill and mentally handicapped people. Instead, such people are to be cared for in their own homes, in small units, or hostels. Thus, many mentally ill patients are now treated in day hospitals, returning to their families in the evening, retaining their links with home, whilst others continue their normal occupations during the day, but go to hostels at night where they can receive supportive therapy. Community psychiatric nurses enable patients to receive some professional support while treatment is given within their own homes.

The policy for care in the community wherever possible rather than in hospital extends to the care of elderly people.

The three groups, elderly, mentally ill and mentally handicapped people, have received special consideration from the Government, following the publication of a report by Sir Roy Griffiths (*Community Care: Agenda for Action*).

A White Paper setting out the Government's policy for community care was published on 14 November 1989. In future, the responsibility for the provision of 'social' care for the groups of people mentioned above will devolve upon local authorities. Such responsibility will be operationalized through local authority social services departments. Provision can and should be made through a 'mixed economy' of services involving the voluntary and private sectors as well as local authority services. The objectives of the policy are:

'to promote the development of domiciliary day and respite services to enable people to live in their own homes wherever feasible and sensible.

to ensure that service providers make practical support for carers a high priority.

to make proper assessment of need and good case management the cornerstone of high quality care.

to promote the development of a flourishing independent
sector alongside good quality public provision.

to clarify the responsibilities of agencies and so make it
easier to hold them to account for their performance.'

Special arrangements are to be made for the mentally
ill, with specific grants to local authorities from 1991–
1992 through Regional Health Authorities. Before each
mentally ill patient is discharged from hospital an assessment is to be made to ascertain both continuing health
care needs and social care. A named person is to be
appointed to ensure that continuing needs are met.

Although special parts of the Register for nurses trained
in mental and mental deficiency (now called mental subnormality) nursing were set up when the Register of Nurses
was established, the Royal Medico-Psychological Association continued to be a recognized body concerned with
the training and examination of nurses in this field. However, in 1947 the Association agreed that it would cease
to carry out this function and that the General Nursing
Council should be the sole body concerned with the
training and examinations for the certificates of mental
and mental deficiency nursing. When this change took
place it was also agreed that nurses who had trained
under the auspices of the Association and held the Association's certificate would be entitled to apply to be registered with the General Nursing Council without
undergoing further training or examinations.

2 The context of nursing and the nurse's role

THE HOSPITAL AND THE COMMUNITY

Chapter 1 indicated in outline how the nursing profession has grown through the ages, sometimes making great strides forward and at other times apparently lost in an age of general indifference to the welfare of the 'common man'. Just as the progress of nursing has reflected the social outlook of a particular age or century, so also have the hospitals and the health and welfare services.

Student nurses at the time of entry to the training school have to adjust themselves to new surroundings and may be somewhat bewildered by the many aspects of hospital life. The student may also have preconceived ideas about the hospital and about nursing, which bear little resemblance to reality. It may be worthwhile, therefore, to consider very briefly the function of the hospital in the community at the present time.

First, the day-to-day function of caring for the sick who lie in the beds in the wards or enter the casualty or out-patient departments. The hospital has to carry on its work day and night. There can be no moment in the 24 hours when the sick are not in need of medical attention and nursing care. This affects not only the medical and nursing staffs but also the ancillary staff and lay workers; porters, orderlies and domestic workers must be available for a 24-hour service, and other departments ancillary to medicine, such as dispensaries, laboratories, X-ray and physiotherapy departments, although these may not always provide a 24-hour service.

Nurse training courses based on Project 2000 recommendations include the study of concepts of health and health promotion, as well as a consideration of the care of people who are ill or disabled. During the course, experience will be gained in the 'community' (e.g. people's homes, hostels, residential homes) as well as in the hospital, so that on registration as a first level nurse the individual is able to work in either setting. Clearly it is worth considering some of the aspects which the hospital and community settings have in common, as well as the differences between them.

Ill health is known to be associated with deprivation, whilst individual behaviour can also affect a person's health status. Students should therefore seek information about the conditions prevailing within the community in which patients live. For example, what is the age/sex structure of the local population? Are there special health features such as a higher than average infantile mortality rate? What is the incidence of conditions such as leukaemia and cancer? Is this higher or lower than the national average? What is the level of homelessness? Is the average wage higher or lower than the UK average? What is the level of unemployment? Is there a local problem in relation to drug or alcohol abuse? What industries predominate in the locality and do any of them pose a special risk to the health of workers or people who live in their vicinity?

Apart from a knowledge of social influence upon health, it is useful to understand the patient's normal background within which he will be nursed, if in the community, or to which he will return on discharge if care is given in hospital. A knowledge of the home background and employment history can help in teaching and counselling patients.

COMMUNITY NURSING

The community nursing service is organized so that each district nurse is responsible for a number of patients. This is frequently based upon a particular family doctor's list. The district nurse is responsible for the nursing assessment of the patient, the identification of priorities, the care plan and its evaluation, and is helped in this work by less highly qualified staff, such as district enrolled nurses and support workers.

By the very nature of the service and its organization, the district nurse does not stay with the patient the whole time but makes a judgement as to the frequency with which professional care is needed. Thus the delivery of care is shared with relatives, friends, or other informal carers if the patient is in a residential home or hostel. Part of the community nurse's role is to teach and support the informal carers. It is important to note that the nurse is a visitor to the patient's home, so the power relationship between the two is rather more equal than is the case in hospital. The nurse can advise on the environment for care but cannot control it as in a hospital. An unsafe environment for care which the nurse is unable to modify would be good grounds for seeking to arrange for the patient's admission to hospital.

A community nurse works within the primary health care team. This comprises the family practitioner, practice nurse, health visitor and community psychiatric nurse, in addition to the district nurse. Occasionally community physiotherapists, occupational therapists and clinical psychologists are available but there are fewer such posts in the community.

HOSPITAL NURSING

Unlike the community nursing service, the hospital nursing service is organized so that nurses are available in the wards over a 24-hour period. Usually there are three shifts of nurses: two to cover the day time and one to cover for the night. Frequently the senior night sister or charge nurse is the manager of the whole site at night. Professionals other than nurses may also work 'unsocial hours'. For example, the accident and emergency department provides a 24-hour service. This will include the provision of X-ray and laboratory facilities and a portering service. Other services, including medical staff, cover by being 'on call' (i.e. they live sufficiently near to the hospital to be there if needed).

One of the main reasons for giving care in the community rather than the hospital, wherever possible, is the problematic nature of the hospital environment from the point of view of patients. Florence Nightingale argued that one objective was that the hospital 'should do the sick no harm'. This is as important an objective today as it always was. It is somewhat ironical to realize that the very place to which the sick may be admitted to help them to get better could be a place of danger. Patients may be at risk of cross-infection or nosocomial infection (transmitted by staff). There are dangerous drugs, harsh disinfectant agents and harmful gases kept within the ward environment. Psychological harm can also arise from the separation of children from their parents and siblings on admission to hospital. Indeed, separation from loved ones can upset adults as well. Patients can be affected by the alien and frightening machinery or the sight of seriously ill patients. Windowless intensive care units can lead to disorientation. The environment in which a patient lives during a hospital stay is controlled by others, not by the patient, and this can be very frustrating.

Hospitals are large and complex organizations to those who are not familiar with them. Their primary purpose is the care and treatment of those who are ill or disabled. In general, the patient's length of stay in hospital is getting shorter and shorter. This is a reflection of Government policy. It is a policy which makes maximum use of the skills of community nurses, and on balance it is better for patients to return to their familiar home environment as soon as possible. Inevitably, however, there are some people whose stay in hospital is prolonged. Such people deserve special consideration because the ward becomes their home. Unfortunately the hospital displays many bureaucratic features and this can lead to institutionalization of long-stay patients. The essence of preventing institutionalization is to provide patients with as much choice as possible. Making the ward as home-like as possible involves running more risks with patients' safety than is permissible in a short-stay ward.

However short the patient's stay, unless it is less than 24 hours, the hospital has to provide 'hotel services' as well as treatment facilities. It can be seen that complex organization is required, involving estate management and maintenance, domestic and catering services, as well as therapeutic services.

Apart from the primary function of the hospital as outlined above, it has other functions which, while secondary are still important. One of these functions is as a training institution. In addition to the training of nurses, the professional education of doctors, radiographers, physiotherapists, midwives and social workers is carried out. Many hospitals take part in the postgraduate training of medical specialists, although not forming part of an undergraduate medical school. Whatever the part played by the individual hospital in professional education, we should not forget the role of the hospitals as health education centres. The aim of treatment is not only to cure or arrest disease but to restore the patient as far as possible to full activity. The motivation of the patient to get well is needed and he must be kept fully informed and counselled so that he can play his part in his own recovery and subsequent welfare.

A further function of the hospital is as an institution for clinical research. Research begins in the laboratory, but discoveries have to be put to the test if they are to have any practical use. In the last century Joseph Lister had theories about safe surgery which would abolish 'hospital gangrene' and septicaemia, from which so many patients died in hospital in spite of surgical skill. If, in the face of much opposition and scepticism, he had not had the courage to put his theories into practice, 'antiseptic surgery', which opened the door to the great surgical advances of the twentieth century, would have been delayed for many years. From the days of Lister's triumphant vindication of his methods, research workers and clinical practitioners have striven to improve on his first great advance in the practice of safe surgery, until in the last decade we have seen the discovery of chemical substances which can control sepsis to a degree undreamed of at the beginning of the century. Present-day methods of surgery are a great advance upon the cruder methods of antiseptic surgery, but Lister's work was the starting point. There are many examples which could be quoted to show that the close collaboration between the laboratory worker and the clinical worker in mitigating the sufferings of mankind is truly a part of the hospital service. The nurse is a part of the clinical research team, a team in which habits of accurate recording, observation and meticulous attention to detail are the first essentials.

A promising development is the recent growth of research into all aspects of nursing, including the quality of nursing care, being undertaken by nurses. A profession should both undertake research into its own practices, and educate its members about that research, so that current practice is based on the results of research. Nursing will then be based on accurate and controlled observation, not opinion.

Given the complexity of the hospital organization and the vulnerability of patients, it is important that all staff act at all times in the best interests of the patients. This also applies when patients are being cared for in the community. It is frequently obvious how staff should behave in order to do their very best for patients. Occasionally, however, there is a dilemma and the best course of action is far from clear. It is in such cases that a code of ethics becomes important.

Both the medical and nursing professions have a code of practice to inform their patients. In addition there are ethical guidelines for clinical research. Each district health authority appoints an ethical committee to consider issues relating to both clinical decisions and research projects.

NURSING ETHICS

Ethics means a code of moral behaviour, and under the term 'ethics of nursing' are included the values and rules of behaviour relating especially to nursing. The word 'nursing' means 'nourishing'; therefore it has come to mean tending and helping all who need it, especially the sick. The object in training nurses is to provide an adequate service to tend the sick, and to help in the preservation and promotion of the health of the community in general.

Those who enter this profession need a real desire to do the work, and must be physically healthy.

Many qualities of personality must be allowed to develop

or mature during the period of training. Kindliness, sympathy and respect for each individual patient, regardless of age, sex, race or social class, are essential qualities for the successful care of the sick person and anxious relatives.

In health education and health promotion activities a nurse must be sensitive to the individual's social and cultural background, so that the advice given fits with the individual's belief system.

A nurse must have personal integrity, so that she can respect a patient's confidence about his private affairs. If told something that ought to be passed on to the nurse in charge or the doctor, because it gives new light on the patient's illness or home situation, the nurse should ask the patient's permission to pass it on. Better still would be to persuade the patient to talk to the sister, charge nurse or doctor personally, since information may be distorted in being passed through a second person. A nurse should be very careful to whom details about the patient's illness or condition are revealed. Nurses should seek the patient's permission before giving information to, say, employers or friends, however much kindly interest these people show.

Importance is rightly placed on complete reliability in carrying out instructions, and punctuality in giving drugs and recording observations. A nurse should be conscientious, so that nursing procedures are carried out properly, even though no one is watching and time is short. A short cut in a sterile procedure may result in cross-infection. Forgetting to remove a patient from a commode or bedpan may lead to the formation of a pressure sore. Patients are unlikely to complain about being forgotten, since most feel a great deal of sympathy with overworked nurses.

The important thing is to maintain an ideal of service to the patient, so that what is best for the patient is foremost at all times. It is also important, however, to have sufficient humility to realize that a nurse does not automatically, and always, know what is best for the patient. Patients should be given a part to play in decisions about their welfare. This not only maintains their self-respect, but also encourages their independence, ready for a return to normal life.

Apart from the qualities already mentioned, a nurse needs to develop emotional maturity, and during the early days of training needs help and support from trained members of staff, so that maturity may be gained healthily.

Ethical problems

There are many episodes which occur in a hospital ward which can upset a nurse emotionally, and a young student needs to be able to discuss these episodes with some mature and trusted person. The student can begin to understand her own emotional reactions and come to terms with them; neither suppressing them on the one hand, nor becoming so upset that she gives up training on the other.

Episodes which may upset a student are, of course very difficult to specify since each student is an individual, and will be affected by different circumstances from another individual.

The death of a patient invariably upsets the nurses in the ward concerned. A young student may be apprehensive before the very first contact with death, and worry about how she will react. The topic should be discussed before the situation arises, so at least she will know what are the right things to do, reducing anxiety in case she should do the wrong thing in a new situation. When a patient has died the nurse should be able to discuss her own reactions to the event. Most people are upset in this situation, and the nurse should be made to realize that this is a normal reaction and not feel guilty that she is 'soft' or 'silly'.

Death of a young patient may be particularly upsetting, and may even bring uncertainties about the nurse's own religious faith. Being able to talk about the situation with a clergyman may help.

News that a patient has an incurable condition can have a similar effect on the nursing staff. Here it is important to let the young student know that these things upset even mature members of staff. They learn, however, to forget their own upset, and put the well-being of the patient or relatives first, and by being helpful to others, tempered with an understanding of how they feel, can come to terms with their own emotions.

In addition, there are problems of conscience which arise, and which each nurse must resolve for herself, in her own way, in the light of her own philosophical beliefs, although talking them over with some trusted person may help.

Obvious problems of conscience are ones thrown up by recent developments in social reform and medicine.

Abortion

Should the nurse participate in the operation of abortion, if she herself strongly disapproves of abortion? If she does disapprove, should this be revealed in her attitude if she nurses a patient who has had an abortion? If she approves of abortion and sees a woman who is unfairly (as she judges) refused one, what should she do if she knows of another doctor who regards abortion more favourably?

Problems of resuscitation

Nowadays it is possible to maintain the heart beat and the exchange of respiratory gases by artificial measures.

Sometimes a nurse may see a patient resuscitated whom she knows will only suffer a great deal if he survives. Although the decision is not the student's the situation may cause great stress to someone asked to nurse the patient.

The problems of abortion, resuscitation and transplant surgery have been well publicized in both the national and nursing press. They are not primarily nursing responsibilities, and most individuals are likely to have made up their minds on these issues in accordance with their own conscience.

However, the nurse may come up against other problems of conscience in day-to-day work on the ward, and these are more likely to be of concern.

For instance, what if the nurse believes a patient should be given full information about his diagnosis and prognosis, and it is being withheld? She can ease her conflict, because the responsibility for this decision is a medical one. But what about this same situation when she is asked point blank by the patient if he is dying, and she knows he is, but the doctor's policy is not to reveal the information to the patient. Should she tell a direct lie? Possible solutions to this problem are suggested in Chapter 16. But although the nurse may cope admirably with the situation, it can still cause some conflict. Or what if she is asked the direct question by a patient, and by a flustered manner and evasiveness leads him to suspect the truth, which is being withheld? Again the nurse will need to be reassured about the whole situation.

The nursing profession has traditionally emphasized that nurses should obey instantly the orders of medical staff and more senior nurses. What if these individuals tell her to do something which she believes is not in the best interests of the patient. Should she argue, or should she obey? This may be something seemingly rather trivial, like being told to go to coffee when a patient has just vomited and needs attention. Nonetheless it can cause conflict for a student, since the ideal of service to the patient and that of respecting the judgement of her seniors, are now incompatible. What if senior nurses treat patients in a way of which she does not approve, and she sees all the other students in the ward following their example? For instance, if an elderly patient is being called by his forename, or 'Dad', without his consent or approval, should she follow the example set? Should she merely maintain her own standards, or should she attempt to change the attitude of other members of staff?

What if a patients is being positively mistreated or neglected? Do her loyalties lie with her colleagues, or should she complain and risk being victimized?

Away from the ward situations, the answers to these problems seem very clear, but issues become very much less clear in the ward situation, where a ward sister, charge nurse or staff nurse is much respected, and has a great deal of knowledge and experience. The individual may feel that there must be some explanation of their conduct which she just does not know. There should be someone to whom she can turn to discuss these problems so that she can see them objectively and then take action as dictated by her own conscience. All nurses, of course, do have a duty to complain if a patient is being mistreated, because a nurse's first duty is to her patient.

Subtle situations may be difficult to judge: when a patient is not being neglected but is just not being treated with the full respect due to a fellow human being, but here again, the first duty of any nurse is to 'nourish' the sick, and this surely includes the patient's mind and spirit, as well as his body.

3 The individual and behaviour related to health care

Modern scientific research has been outstandingly successful in the prevention and/or treatment of most of those diseases that, in the early part of the present century, were responsible for the low life expectancy of people born into what are today's developed countries. Those successes have dramatically changed the demographic structure of Western society; however, in this chapter we will concentrate upon the UK only. Here, with the wide availability of contraception the proportion of young people in the population is falling and will continue to do so over the next decade. At the same time the proportion of elderly people (over 65 years) is rising. In particular, it is the proportions of those over 75 and those over 85 which are set to increase dramatically over the next two decades.

Apart from infant mortality, accidents are the main health problem until middle age, when cancer, myocardial infarction and stroke take over as the major causes of death and morbidity (Lee and Franks, 1980). Elderly people are presenting with health problems which cause enormous morbidity and demands on care. Over the age of 75, health problems increase and apart from those mentioned above there are three conditions affecting this age group which make particularly high levels of demand upon health services: dementia, osteoporosis and osteoarthritis.

The occurrence of accidents, some forms of cancer, and cardiovascular disease appear to be related, in part at least, to individual behaviour. The public health measures so successful in dealing with the diseases of the past have been institutionalized and are now part of routine measures taken more or less for granted within our society. Attention is now focused upon the individual's responsibility for health; the methods used to promote health need to be much more subtle. Education, attitude change, support and encouragement of self-help activities are needed to help people to incorporate health promoting behaviour into their daily routines.

In relation to the promotion and maintenance of health, prevention has been grouped into three types:

1. *Primary prevention* is action which has as its goal the prevention of disease or disability before it occurs. Examples include the immunization of individuals against specific infectious diseases.
2. *Secondary prevention* is action taken once a disease or health problem has occurred and is designed to detect and treat the problem at the earliest possible moment.
3. *Tertiary prevention* occurs when an individual is actively suffering from a health problem, has a chronic disease or a residual disability. Action here is directed at avoiding the progression of the disease or the occurrence of complications; for example, prevention of infection in individuals who have diabetes mellitus.

The importance of the prevention of health problems appears so self-evident that a naïve view would suppose that all the health professionals need to do is to tell people about the dangers and how to avoid them and all will be well. Clearly things are not that simple but only one or two examples of why the issues may be problematic can be included here.

In primary prevention one of the problems is to motivate people to take action against health problems many years before there is any apparent risk at all. For example, eating patterns established in childhood may lead to obesity and high cholesterol levels in mid-life, increasing the risk of coronary heart disease. Smoking cigarettes in adolescence may lead to bronchitic problems or worse in mid-life. When one is young, the idea of health problems occurring at the age of 50 years or so seems such a long time in the future that it is difficult to relate it to oneself at all. The issue is complicated by the fact that the relationship between the behaviour mentioned above and health problems is complex. One is increasing the probability of a disease occurring rather than ensuring its inevitable onset. Individuals are frequently able to counter evidence on the link between smoking and lung cancer, for example, by citing a relative who smoked all his life and lived happily to the age of 85 or so. Clearly it is important to get parents to promote healthy routines in their offspring at a young age. It is also often the case that the preventive action is less attractive than the risky behaviour. Furthermore, in the case of immunization, the effects of the injections against some diseases may cause great discomfort or side-effects and knowledge of this may act as a deterrent to receiving immunization.

Secondary prevention requires the individual to seek medical help at the earliest possible moment. There are many reasons why an individual may delay going to the doctor. Unfortunately the individual who suspects he may have cancer frequently delays through anxiety, which may be enough to lead to denial.

A model of how an individual's health beliefs may influence him in seeking help when feeling ill was proposed by Rosenstock in 1966. This model describes the decision to seek medical help as a function of (1) the individual's perception of his own susceptibility to the illness, and (2) his beliefs as to the seriousness of the consequences of the illness. These, taken together, are said to affect the individual's readiness to act. Even so, he must identify the action as readily available and that, if carried out, it will be beneficial. A triggering factor is still required, according to Rosenstock, and this results from inter-personal events which are unspecified in the model. Whilst this model has been criticized and is somewhat vague, it does underline the complexity of behaviour in relation to health.

Turning now to tertiary prevention, a problem occurs due to the nature of some of the actions required to prevent complications. Frequently, individuals with chronic conditions, need to carry out time-consuming actions faithfully day after day in an unremitting way. There is no holiday from injections of insulin or watching one's diet for the person with insulin-dependent diabetes mellitus. Other conditions may make even heavier demands upon the sufferer's life-style. For example, the person in renal failure must carry out dialysis two to three times a week. 'Tedium' is a term which has been used to describe the stress that occurs when a heavy demand is made on the individual for a taxing routine for which there is no let up (Lundman et al, 1988).

HEALTH PROMOTION AIMS AND METHODS

The importance of prevention has been accepted by nurses since the teaching of Florence Nightingale in the nine-teenth century. However, during the period from the end of the nineteenth century until comparatively recently, the individual with the major role in this area was the health visitor. It is now recognized that prevention is an important component in the role of all nurses, and recent guidance from the nursing statutory bodies includes health promotion and health education as important components of the syllabuses leading to first level registration. This, to a large extent, is based on the World Health Organization's proclaimed policy of health for all by the year 2000 (WHO, 1986).

Perhaps we should first indicate what we mean by the terms 'health education' and 'health promotion'. Health education is a term which has been in use for some considerable length of time. It refers to educational activities which have a goal in the areas of primary, secondary or tertiary prevention. Health promotion is something rather more positive. 'Health' is difficult to define and probably means different things to different people. However, it is generally accepted that it means more than the mere absence of disease.

Coutts and Hardy (1985) made the following statements about health:

1. Health means different things to different people.
2. Health means more than the absence of disease or infirmity.
3. Health equals adaptability.
4. Health optimum varies.
5. Health is necessary for the purpose of life and adds to the quality of life.

Therefore, in engaging in health promotion we are helping individuals to achieve their potential.

The goals of health education and promotion were summarized by Levin (Levin et al, 1977). They are to:

1. Contribute to self-fulfillment of individuals and promote their well-being, as they define it.
2. Enhance the ability of people to cope effectively with

health promotion, health maintenance and illness control.

3. Reduce undesired risks of disease and illness.
4. Help people maintain personal and civil integrity whilst receiving health care.
5. Create more active individual and community participation in the health system by increasing (1) personal competence in self-care, and (2) social skills in working within the formal health system.

Just as individuals have beliefs about health which influence their behaviour in relation to health and illness, so do those who advocate health education and promotion activities on the part of professionals. These beliefs are (1) that personal or collective behaviour affect health status, and (2) that it is possible to change the health related behaviour of individuals or communities by planned intervention.

Within the general area of health education there are several different types and styles of activity, depending partly upon an individual's professional background and beliefs about the most effective and ethical way of changing health related behaviour.

1. *Information-giving* This involves the use of planned information presented in an interesting and easily understood way. This method leaves people to decide for themselves what use they will make of such information. There is also a suggestion that for some people this method assumes that individuals are 'empty vessels' to be filled with information.
2. *Educational method.* Here, theories of learning and teaching techniques are employed. It is recognized that not only is it important to address the knowledge of the individual but also his or her emotions, since these have an important influence upon health related

behaviour. Methods of teaching employed include group discussion, experiential learning and other student centred styles. The aim of such methods includes helping the individual to develop decision making skills and to clarify his or her feelings about health.

3. *Propagandizing*. All professional communication media may be employed in this approach: for example, television and cinema advertisements, documentary programmes, advertisements in newspapers and magazines, magazine articles, and the use of radio and television 'serials'. Given the enormous financial implications of such approaches, this method is clearly usually only available to government or government-sponsored organizations.

4. *Enabling strategies*. This approach assumes that the individual wishes to be active in promoting his own health but needs the necessary information and opportunity to make informed choices. The health professional deliberately takes the non-directive approach. Individuals or self-help groups are stimulated to identify their own health concerns and needs and to identify for themselves the appropriate action.

5. *Political action*. Here, it is believed that many health problems relate to the broader environment and cannot be solved by individual behaviour. Thus, political action is necessary to bring about environmental and societal change.

THE TEACHING PROCESS

A thorough exploration of the issues relating to teaching and learning is well beyond the scope of this book; many textbooks have been devoted to these topics. For health education and promotion activities the individual needs a knowledge of learning theories, education techniques and theories, and theoretical and practical knowledge of attitude formation and change. However, a lack of formal expertize in teaching should not deter the nurse from health promotion activities. Indeed, it has been said that nurses are continually teaching, whether they recognize it or not. This is why so much concern has been expressed at the incidence of smoking within the nursing profession. The smell of smoking on the clothes of a nurse may well be teaching patients that it is acceptable to smoke, since the nurse could be expected to exemplify healthy behaviour.

The first stage in health education/promotion is assessment of the individual or group. It will be assumed here that the focus of concern is an individual rather than a group.

Assessment

Assessment should ascertain the person's developmental stage, any potential difficulties for communication (such as deafness), the language they understand, the level of anxiety, their alertness and any pain. Excessive levels of anxiety or pain will interfere with the individual's ability to learn. Sometimes the use of denial as a defence mechanism also interferes with the individual's ability to remember what is taught. For example, if the person is employing denial as a means of coping with body image change following colostomy, any teaching about colostomy management is likely to be ineffective.

An important factor in ensuring the effectiveness of teaching is the recipient's readiness to learn. Motivation makes all the difference between success and failure. Usually, patients, clients and informal carers are well motivated to learn because the issue is one of supreme importance to their future. In addition, nurses often have greater opportunities for teaching than other health professionals because of the type of nurse—patient/client relationship which develops. Occasionally there are problems when the patient expects one type of information and the nurse is intending to teach something else. This should be detected by careful assessment so that mutual expectations can be exchanged.

Action

Having assessed the patient/client, the next step is to plan the teaching. First, the goals, aims and objectives are identified. These should be expressed in a clear, patient-centred way. For example, what is it that the patient/client will know, feel or do as a result of the teaching? Then, taking account of the patient's previous knowledge, the method to be used is identified. Except in the case of practical skill teaching the choice is really between the fairly straightforward information protocol or a more interactive counselling style. Written information may also be used.

Information giving

Let us first discuss the straighforward information protocol. The information needs to be planned out using a format in which the reason for giving information is explained first, followed by the most important information to be given (Ley and Spelman, 1967). The most important information relates to the goal which has been identified. Simple, clear language should be chosen so that the individual has no difficulty in understanding it. The exposition should proceed logically from point to point. It is better to plan to give only short pieces of information at a time, unless it can be backed up with written information. This helps the individual to remember what they have been told. Finally, plan to summarize and repeat the main point, inviting questions.

It is important to ensure a quiet environment, and as far as possible a period of time which will be interruption-free, before approaching the patient and sitting down to talk.

Counselling style

This takes account of some of the principles of therapeutic communication. It ensures the commitment of the patient/client/carer to the course of action rather better than does straight information-giving. However, a greater degree of skill is required on the part of the nurse. Counselling can be said to include several phases.

Facilitation

Here the nurse talks to the patient and listens in a warm empathetic and non-directive way. This develops a trusting relationship.

Transition

Here the patient is encouraged to open up as far as possible. The nurse asking the patient relevant questions to help this process. Self-disclosure on the nurse's part may be used to encourage the patient to be open as well. The nurse needs to demonstrate interest in the patient and genuineness. The purpose of this phase is to come to a point where the problem is defined jointly.

Action

Strategies to deal with the problem are jointly planned. In this phase the nurse may use confrontation as a strategy;

for example, if the patient agrees a course of action but it is known that he has agreed many times in the past but never fulfilled promises.

Finally, when the issue has been explored and commitment to a course of action is obtained, the stage of termination is reached.

It can be seen how this method contrasts with the previous method. Here there is no possibility of thinking out beforehand a plan of what one will say. Instead, a clear identification of the objectives and an ability to use the cues given by the patient is needed. Cues steer the interaction toward the objective or to an abandonment of the attempt. Clearly the patient is much more in command of this situation.

Practical skills

The nurse frequently needs to teach a practical skill to a patient or carer. For example, a diabetic patient or the carer may need to be taught to administer an insulin injection, to test urine, and to test blood glucose levels. It is necessary to plan out what is to be done in the teaching session and how to do it. The nurse needs not only to be proficient but to recognize those key points in a skill which require emphasis and possibly repetitive demonstration.

The patient/carer should be given a description of the procedure before watching it so that he is in a state of readiness and knows what to look for. A running commentary is then needed while the procedure is slowly carried out and the main points are emphasized. Finally, there should be a summary of the main points and a chance for questions.

Eventually, after several demonstrations, the individual

will start to practice the skill and here, too, the nurse needs to keep up a running commentary, praising and encouraging good points and correcting where necessary. This process is repeated until the individual is proficient.

Evaluation

Evaluation of the teaching can be related back to the goals and objectives. The patient/client/carer should be able to demonstrate that he now has the knowledge or has done something as specified in the goal. Ensuring that a goal relating to 'feeling' has been achieved is not quite so straightforward. It is possible to ask the patient, for example, how did you feel about having the injection? The other possibility is to use a published scale, for example an anxiety scale, to identify if the person's anxiety has been reduced as a result of the intervention.

STRESS AND COPING

Over the past decade stress as a concept has received a great deal of attention within the nursing and psychological literature. It is now generally accepted that a person's perception that he is ill acts as a stressor, whilst pain and other symptoms increase the stress which is experienced. Admission to hospital may also act as a stressor, depending upon the individual. It has been known for some time that a surgical procedure provokes physiological stress quite apart from any psychological effects it has. Clearly, stress is a concept which deserves discussion in a textbook on nursing.

Stress has been defined as arising out of the individual's appraisal of a mismatch between demands made on him and his ability to cope (Clarke, 1984). This is the definition being adopted for the purposes of this book and we should note that it is a psychological definition. It is important to bear the definition in mind since the word 'stress' may be used very loosely in every day conversation. Even between scientific textbooks the concept may be defined differently. Although the definition adopted for this book is a psychological one, this is not intended to deny the importance of the physiological component of stress and it is to this that we turn first.

Physiological aspects of stress

The major figure in research on the physiology of stress is Hans Selye (1956). He described both the physiological component of stress and the sequence of events set in train in responding to a stressor. He called this sequence of events the general adaptation syndrome (GAS).

Let us first examine at least some of the physiological components of stress. In responding to a stressor, both the autonomic nervous system (ANS) and the endocrine system have a large part to play. The ANS, and in particular the sympathetic system, not only has a role in the stimulation of effector tissue such as plain muscle, but also stimulates the adrenal medulla to release adrenaline and noradrenaline (these two hormones are known as catecholamines) into the bloodstream. These hormones enhance the effect of ANS stimulation. Whilst there is little doubt that many hormones are involved in the response to a stressor, the role of the glucocorticoids secreted by the adrenal cortex is paramount.

The combined effects of the ANS catecholamine release and glucocorticoid release are of significance in the nursing of patients and so these effects will be briefly listed:

1. The blood pressure and pulse rate are raised and the cardiac output is increased.

2. The central nervous system is activated via the reticular activating system.
3. Blood sugar is raised.
4. Body fluid is conserved.
5. Blood coagulability is increased.
6. The inflammatory response may be suppressed.
7. There is a redistribution of blood to heart, muscle and brain.

Clearly, most of these effects are beneficial in the perioperative period. If the response is prolonged, however, some effects may be problematic during the postoperative period. For example, the increase in blood coagulability may predispose to deep vein thrombosis and hence to pulmonary emboli. The depressed inflammatory response, combined with breakdown of glycogen and then protein to maintain the blood glucose, can lead to poor wound healing and possible infection. It can thus be seen how important it is to prevent stress levels from rising and/or from being prolonged in patients in general, and in patients undergoing operations in particular. One way of preventing stress levels from rising is to give appropriate preoperative information to patients. This will be discussed further later in this chapter.

The general adaptation syndrome described by Selye has three phases:

1. The stage of alarm
2. The stage of resistance
3. The stage of exhaustion.

Fortunately, the process usually ends during the stage of resistance and the individual adapts to the stressor, which then has no further effects. However, an individual who enters the stage of exhaustion has indeed exhausted the body's energy resources and ability to cope. Death may ensue. Care should be aimed at reinforcing the body's homeostatic and energy resources to prevent the stage of exhaustion. This stage may be reached in relation to extremely severe stressors, or additional stressors occurring when the body is already coping with earlier stressors.

Psychological aspects of stress

Whilst a consideration of the physiological aspects of stress is crucial within health care, psychological aspects are equally important, especially when considering stress in everyday life and its relationship to health. In the Western world most of the stressors which we perceive daily as making demands on us are psychological in nature. According to our definition, these lead to stress if we feel unable to cope. We have already discussed the physiological components of stress. How appropriate is it for our blood pressure, pulse rate and blood sugar level to rise when we perceive, for example, that work demands are greater than we believe we can cope with? Clearly the physiological response is not going to help us to work harder; nor will it help in dealing in a more appropriate way with a difficult colleague. Indeed, a deliberately difficult colleague may identify the signs of increased blood pressure and feel a sense of reward for difficult behaviour, leading to still further problems.

Stress and health

It is the very inappropriateness of physiological responses in many stressful circumstances which has led to the view that the onset of ill health may actually be associated with stress in the recent past. An obvious example is the condition of hypertension (consistently high blood pressure), since blood pressure rises in stress. It will be recalled that hypertension is a risk factor for coronary heart disease. Many of the group of conditions classified as psychosomatic have been frequently cited as being associated with stress.

Some interesting work by Holmes and Rahe (1967) went further than this. They identified a list of events which occur regularly from time to time in everyone's life and then asked groups of individuals to estimate the severity of such incidents in terms of stress. As a result, each instance was assigned a number of 'life-change units,' as Holmes and Rahe called them. It was then possible to ask people to identify the instances to which they had been subjected during the past year and to add up all the resulting life-change units. Studies in which this has been done show that the higher the number of total life-change units in the preceding 6–12 months, the more likely the individual is to become ill.

In the light of research suggesting that stress increases the probability that illness will occur, one of the health promotion activities offered to patients, clients and carers is teaching within the area of stress control. Such teaching may concentrate on getting the individual to perceive stressful events differently so that they are no longer felt as being stressful. Another group of stress control methods which can be taught include those which counter the physiological components of stress, for example, relaxation and transcendental meditation. These reduce blood pressure, pulse and respiratory rates and bring about skeletal muscular relaxation.

Emotion, defence mechanisms and stress

Clearly, psychological events may make heavy demands on an individual's capacity for coping, and our definition of stress incorporates this view. Whilst physiological views of stress are necessary, they are no longer sufficient to account for all situations in which stress occurs. Physiological explanations of stress deal with stressors such as infection, trauma, poisons and extreme environmental temperatures, and describe the process of adaptation to these stressors. Such a view cannot account, for example, for the individual's experience of the death of a spouse, failure in an examination or rejection at job interview. Nor does the physiological view of stress account for people's experience in extremely impoverished environments with lack of stimulation. We all know, too, that conditions associated for stress with one individual may have little or no effect upon another person. For example, rejection at a job interview may be extremely stressful for one person but of no significance to another. Psychological views of stress take account of these factors.

As well as acknowledging the importance of stressors of a psychological type, we need to consider psychological issues in coping with stressors. Furthermore, the relationship between emotion and stress requires some explanation.

Frequently, the individual's experience of stress is in terms of an emotion, such as fear. People may tell you they are angry, upset, depressed or anxious in response to a demanding situation. Depression, for example, is so common in bereavement that we may well believe someone to be abnormal if they do not appear depressed. Similarly, anxiety is extremely common in stressful situations. Anxiety frequently accompanies the sympathetic nervous system arousal which is part of the physiological component of stress.

However, the relationship between stress and negative emotional states is extremely complex. We have mentioned that negative emotions are aroused by stressors. What we have not said yet is that negative emotions can act as stressors. This may happen when threat or demand has not been recognized at a conscious level. Negative emotion is experienced (usually fear and/or anxiety), and this acts as a stressor. The fact that negative emotions have this complex relationship with stress means that they can exacerbate a problem. For example, let us suppose that someone experiences anxiety on finding a lump in their breast. The perception of the lump and all that this may mean in terms of coping triggers anxiety. However, the anxiety can not only act as an additional stressor but may be severe enough to actually interfere with the coping needed, that is, going to the general practitioner as soon as possible. This complex relationship between stress and emotion has been addressed in the research of Lazarus (Lazarus and Launier, 1978). He has concentrated particularly upon coping and shown that coping strategies employed by an individual may have two functions: (1) the regulation of emotional responses, and (2) the regulation of behaviour aimed at mitigating the stressor.

Many studies researching into stress have measured levels of negative emotions as an indicator of stress. This is particularly the case in studies of patients. Measurement of anxiety is comparatively easy and anxiety scales are frequently employed to identify the effectiveness of interventions designed to reduce stress.

Relaxation techniques are aimed at the regulation of emotional responses through the regulation of sympathetic nervous system arousal. It should be obvious that, if effective, such measures prevent stress levels rising and allow the individual to begin to cope with the stressor, using intellectual and behavioural strategies.

Coping strategies which may be employed by the individual as a defence against high levels of negative emotions may be at the unconscious level. These are the defence mechanisms described by Freud (Colman and Hamman,

1974). From the dozen or so defence mechanisms included in the work of Freudian psychologists, just one, denial, will be mentioned here. Denial is an important defence mechanism used by patients with physical conditions and so it is frequently encountered in clinical nursing. It should be remembered, however, that patients will use other defence mechanisms as well.

Within the psychiatric and psychological literature, defence mechanisms are frequently evaluated very negatively. They are regarded as long-term blocks preventing the individual from living life to the full. However, explorations of denial in particular and its role in coping with severe stress associated with devastating events (for example, bereavement, life threatening conditions) reveals that defence mechanisms may have a positive function. They appear to act as 'filters', preventing the individual from having to handle too much disabling information at a given time (Parkes, 1972). Denial acts as if it is buying the individual time during which personal resources can be built up in order to face and cope with a major and devastating stressor. However, it must be emphasized that defence mechanisms, by definition, are unconscious and that the individual is certainly not using them consciously.

Denial has been described as a stage both in the process of coping with our own impending death (Kubler-Ross, 1969) and in bereavement (Parkes, 1972).

The use of denial and other defence mechanisms was described in a study of 21 women with breast cancer over a 2-year period (Gyllensköld, 1982). What was interesting in this study by a clinical psychologist was the way in which defence mechanisms were used by the women during a series of interviews with the researcher. These were carried out at critical points in the women's total experience. Defence mechanisms were used in a labile way, being employed one moment and not the next. Partial denial of the disease was employed. Denial might, for instance, be used when interacting with relatives but not with doctors. Patients were consciously afraid of emotions, but Gyllensköld believes that energy locked up in maintaining the defence mechanism could, if released by crying, be used to cope more constructively with the disease.

From the nursing point of view, nurses should be aware when defence mechanisms are being used because some kinds of information are useless if offered to the patient at that time. Similarly, awareness of the moment when the patient ceases to use denial is important since a great deal of empathic support will then be required if the patient is not to be completely overwhelmed.

Other types of coping

Clearly, the logical way of coping with demands is to do something that will help to reduce the demand: for example, to delegate if work demands are very heavy. But not all situations can be dealt with in that way; in some circumstances, in coming to terms with loss for example, little direct action is possible. Here, coping focused upon emotional states is useful.

Many situations, however, benefit from the individual developing a strategy beforehand to plan how to cope when demand occurs. In some senses we could be said to use this method to cope with the demand of examinations. However, in order to plan coping one needs information. Nurses can help patients to develop coping strategies by giving them information prior to nursing procedures, diagnostic investigations, surgical operations, and so on.

A stressor that has not so far been mentioned is the perception that one has no control over a situation. This appears to be a very potent stressor both in man and animals. It is a stressor which is relevant both to patients and their friends and families. Loss of control is experienced when a diagnosis is not known, and particularly when the prognosis is not known. In addition, a great deal of control is given up to others when a person enters hospital as a patient. There are two ways in which nurses can help the patient suffering from loss of control. One is by giving as much information as possible; this helps to make events more predictable. The other is by giving as much choice to the patient as possible in areas which concern him.

Stress related aspects of nursing care

Amongst the caseload of patients cared for by the district nurse there are invariably individuals who have been discharged from hospital. Stress initiated in relation to impending discharge from hospital will be discussed later. Nurses working in the community will readily understand that to adjust back to life at home requires effort on the patient's part. For some, this effort may be considerable. It involves taking increased responsibility for managing their own condition; alternatively, it means being dependent upon informal carers, with intermittent visits from the district nursing service. Whatever the shortcomings of being in hospital, there is the security of knowing that professionals are readily available day and night in the ward. On discharge, the individual may at first feel very insecure and frightened that things may go wrong and that the family will be unable to cope.

Since the policy is to care for people within the community rather than hospital, wherever possible, it is the community nurse who provides a great deal of the care for those with chronic conditions. There are many demands on patients' coping reserves in this situation. These have been listed by Strauss et al (1984) and include:

1. The long-term nature of the condition and the uncertainty associated with prognosis in many cases.
2. The intrusion of the condition upon the life-style of patients, relatives, friends and the household routine.
3. Social isolation is frequently the consequence, not only for the sufferer but for the family and friends.
4. Prescribed regimens must be carried out. These may leave little time or energy for other more enjoyable activities.
5. The condition may get worse and require further adjustment.

Over and above these issues, some chronic diseases and conditions have stigmatizing elements or other extremely negative connotations, for example, acquired immune deficiency syndrome (AIDS), cancer, or when a patient is known to be dying. This makes the load harder to bear for patient and carers alike. Considerable personal resources are needed by all concerned in coping. Supportive help from the district nursing service may make all the difference between coping and not coping.

Clearly the community nurse must be constantly alert for potential and actual stressors affecting both patients and informal carers. Additional stress factors occur when patients are admitted to hospital, and it is to this situation that we now turn.

Stress and the hospital patient

A little imagination tells us that being admitted to hospital is a critical event within an individual's life. Research confirms that it is indeed perceived as a source of threat by many patients. It not only means that the person is actually or potentially ill, but that the illness is such that it cannot be dealt with by professionals in the community.

Hospital admission causes temporary separation from family and friends and a disruption to the individual's normal social and professional roles. The hospital environment is strange to most people who are not themselves health professionals. Furthermore, it is an environment under the control of people other than patients. However, we must not neglect the highly individual nature of people and it is certainly the case that some individuals admitted for long-awaited operations may respond very positively to admission. For most, however, it is a negative event.

It would be a very sad comment upon our health services if the whole of the patient's stay in hospital was continually and uniformly characterized by high stress levels which were reflected by negative emotional states. Fortunately, a study carried out by Wilson-Barnett and Carrigy (1978) suggests that negative emotional states are at a high level only at certain points within a hospital stay. The study monitored the emotional reactions of 202 medical patients in two hospitals. Anxiety and depression levels were measured each day during the whole of each patient's hospital stay. High scores were found on the day of admission, the day of a special test and, in one of the hospitals, at weekends. Low scores were found in one hospital on the day of discharge but not in the other.

Such information can help nurses to target more precisely their intervention techniques to help patients in their coping. For example, special attention to admission procedures and the provision of clear information to assist patients to cope with settling into the strange environment and routine will be helpful. Wilson-Barnett (1978) showed that giving information relevant to a special test helped to reduce patients' anxiety levels. Furthermore, she showed that the more disturbing the special test was to a patient, the greater the effect of giving information.

It has long been the case that schools of nursing have taught nurses to start a procedure by 'telling the patient what you are going to do' but research by Johnson et al (1978) has shown that this is totally inadequate in helping patients to cope with procedures. Instead, patients need to know how the procedure will affect them, how they will feel, and what they can do to help. The provision of information to an individual about the procedure to be undergone is a skilled activity. It requires careful assessment of the information needs of the individual concerned, and careful planning and timing.

Information is needed in advance so that patients can come to terms with what is going to happen and to rehearse their coping strategy. On the other hand, timing of information should not be so long before the event that the patient has forgotten all about it by the time the procedure is carried out. Another important factor is the careful selection of the information which is given. All information should be given from the patient's point of view. What the patient needs is to know how the procedure will affect him, how to prepare for it, what it will feel like, what the after-effects will be whether he will need to rest afterwards, and so on.

The research by Johnson and co-workers mentioned above has shown the effectiveness of what they call 'sensory information' in helping the patient. In relation to surgery, such information has been shown to increase recovery times of patients, but its importance has also been demonstrated in medical patients.

OTHER COMMUNICATION SKILLS

By now it should be apparent how important good teaching and interactional skills are in nursing. What has not been mentioned so far is the importance of listening and non-verbal communication.

One of the best ways in which a nurse can support a patient, relative or carer during a difficult period is to show empathy. Empathy can be conveyed by listening actively. It can also be conveyed by other aspects of non-verbal behaviour; for example, sitting by the person, maintaining good eye contact, holding the individual's hand, putting one's arm around the patient's shoulder. In short, 'being with' the other individual in all senses.

4 Organization of nursing care: the nursing process

Organization of care for patients/clients in the community is based upon each nurse or health visitor taking responsibility for a number of 'cases' which is then known as the caseload. The caseload may be geographical, the nurse or health visitor seeing all individuals within a locality who are referred for their services. Alternatively the community nurses and health visitors may be 'general practitioner attached'. Here, the general practitioner's list becomes the source of referrals to the other members of the primary health care team. Since health visitors, community psychiatric nurses and community nurses for mentally handicapped people require qualifications beyond that of first level registration, further discussion here will be limited to that of district nursing. Currently, district nurses do receive specialist post-basic training. It is unclear whether this will remain necessary for nurses trained through the Project 2000 courses. Even now, some registered general nurses are employed in the community before taking up a place on a training course.

As indicated above, each trained district nurse is responsible for a caseload of patients, but does not necessarily carry out personally all the nursing care required by these patients. The initial nursing assessment, goal setting, care planning and evaluation are the responsibility of the trained district nurse. Day to day care, however, is frequently delegated, as appropriate, to less highly qualified nurses; for example registered general nurses, district enrolled nurses, enrolled nurses, health care assistants. Care is also carried out by informal carers between visits by the district nursing staff. Informal carers include friends and relatives of the patient, voluntary workers, and non-nursing staff in residential hostels and homes. Clearly, informal carers may require some training in simple nursing procedures and will also require a great deal of support. This is all a part of the district nurse's role.

The nursing role includes monitoring the condition of each patient, giving drugs and treatment on time, preventing the occurrence of complications, and ensuring that each patient is cared for in terms of his physical, psychological and social needs. To do this requires the determination of priorities between competing patient needs and the organization of the nursing team to meet those needs.

The way in which the role of the nurse is defined affects the way in which care is organized and given. In turn, the organizational structure in which nursing occurs affects the selection of activities a nurse carries out with a patient, the priority she gives to those activities and the way in which she gives nursing care. For this reason it is important that ideas about what nursing is are made explicit so that their influence on what is done can be examined and restrictive views may be discarded.

Until comparatively recently, views about the nature of nursing and the role of the nurse were given little attention once a nurse had completed the training. It is now recognized that these issues are crucial to the quality of the nursing service which is offered to a patient. For example, the way the nurse defines his or her role influences the following issues:

1. *The priority given to particular patients within a caseload*. For example, if a nurse defines her role as helping

patients to 'get better' he or she may assign low priority to the care of a dying patient.

2. *The type of nursing problem identified*. For example, if the nurse defines the role as limited to carrying out nursing procedures, the patient's need for information may be ignored.

3. *The nursing intervention suggested*. For example, a nurse who defines the role narrowly may focus upon the patient's current problem, such as adapting to colostomy, and fail to give health education about the dangers of smoking.

The realization that important aspects of nursing care have been devalued in the recent past has led to the development of nursing models. These take as their starting point a statement of nursing ideals and beliefs. The adoption of one particular model as an explicit statement relating to the role of the nurse clarifies for all concerned the priorities being adopted by the nurse who is accountable for patient care.

Most nursing models were developed in the USA but one of the most popular in the UK was developed by three nurses working in Scotland (Roper et al, 1980).

Perhaps the most influential nurse since Florence Nightingale is Virginia Henderson. There is little doubt that the development of nursing models is a result of her careful analysis of the function of nursing. Her (1964) definition of the role of the nurse is still relevant today.

> 'The unique function of the nurse is to assist the individual, sick or well, in the performance of those activities contributing to health or its recovery (or to peaceful death) that he would perform unaided if he had the necessary strength, will or knowledge. And to do them in such a way as to help him gain independence as rapidly as possible. This aspect of her work, this part of her function, she initiates

and controls; of this she is master. In addition, she helps
the patient to carry out the therapeutic plan as initiated
by the physician. She also, as a member of the medical
team, helps other members, as they in turn help her, to
plan and carry out the total programme whether it be for
the improvement of health, or the recovery from illness or
support in death.'

NURSING MODELS

Unlike the use of the term 'model' in science, nursing models
are 'sets of ideas about people and nursing which can be
used as guides for the planning and delivery of nursing
care' (Aggleton and Chalmers, 1986). They are useful
precisely because they make explicit the value system
underlying the view of nursing held by the author of the
model. The value of such models would be enormous if a
specific model were chosen individually for use with each
patient according to the patient's personality, history and
circumstances. However, such a method would demand
that nurses were so familiar with all models that they
could share some of their precepts with patients. What
has become the norm in this country is for the ward
staff, and/or the education department to choose to use a
specific model within a ward, department or hospital.
More freedom is available for district nurses to choose a
model for care because they have their own caseload but,
even here, it is usually the case that each district nurse
and her team chooses just one model to use with all
patients they see.

There are quite a number of different models available
for use, although a smaller number are usually dealt with
in nurse education courses and a smaller number still are
in common use. Models can be classified in various ways.
For example, Riehl and Roy (1980) classify models as
follows:

- Developmental models
    Peplau model
    Systems in change model of Chrisman and Fowler
- System models
    Neuman health care systems model
    Roy adaptation model
    Johnson behavioural system model
    Orem self-care model
    Martha Rogers science of unitary man model
- Interaction models
    Riehl interaction model
    Priesner model for the nurse therapist

In addition to these models, which are all included in Riehl and Roy's book, we can add King's systems model, which is an interactionist model (Aggleton and Chalmers, 1990); Roper, Logan and Tierney's model, a developmental model; and Clark's (1985) model for health visiting. Undoubtedly there are other models for nurses but those listed here are those included in standard textbooks and papers.

It is worth noting that both the Neuman health care systems model and the Roy adaptation model centre around the concept of stress, whilst Clark's (1985) model for health visiting depends on the concept of coping. Nursing care based upon an understanding of stress and coping was discussed in Chapter 3.

The remainder of this section will be concerned with the two most popular models used in the UK in general adult nursing.

Roper, Logan and Tierney's model of nursing

This model focuses upon 12 activities of daily living (ADL), for each of which there is a dependence—independence continuum.

- Maintaining a safe environment
- Communicating
- Breathing
- Eating and drinking
- Eliminating
- Personal cleansing and dressing
- Controlling body temperature
- Mobilizing
- Working and playing
- Expressing sexuality
- Sleeping
- Dying

Factors said to influence the individual in relation to these ADL are physical, psychological, sociocultural, environmental and politico-economic.

A further component of the model is the individual's life span, which clearly affects the way in which the individual carries out the ADL, both in health and illness.

Assessment is carried out in each of the daily living activities, identifying the patient's/client's dependence—independence on each dimension. Influences to which the individual is subject are also noted. Goal setting, care planning and evaluation of care also focus in turn on each daily living activity for which the individual is not fully independent.

This model is undoubtedly the most popular one within the UK at the time of writing. The main reasons for its popularity are its freedom from jargon and its ease of use. It is appropriate to a wide variety of people with physical health problems and it ensures reasonably comprehensive nursing care. Compared with most of the other models listed above, it is fairly simple. This is a valuable attribute if the formulation of goals of care and the identification of nursing problems are to be shared with patients and/or their families.

Orem's self-care model

The concept of self-care is central to this model. Self-care consists of those activities which, carried out by each individual in full health, maintain life, health and well-being. Such activities are learned. ('Self-care agency' is the term used in Orem's writing but as such terminology is alien to the UK it will not be used in this book.)

Orem lists six basic self-care abilities practised in health which she terms universal self-care demands. These are:

- Adequate intake of air, water and food
- Adequate excretion of waste products
- A balance between rest and activity: mental and physical
- Optimization of social interaction and solitude
- Avoidance and prevention of hazards to life and well-being
- Feeling and being normal, thereby avoiding stress

Three further types of self-care needs occur in illness. These are called health deviation self-care needs and they are of the following types:

- Relating to changes in body structure
- Relating to changes in physical function
- Relating to changes in behaviour

If self-care demands or needs cannot be met by the individual then 'self-care deficit' occurs. It is these self-care deficits which are the concern of carers, whether informal or professional. If the patient is completely unable to fulfil any of the self-care needs then nursing is said to be 'wholly compensatory'. Where the individual can carry out some, but not all, self-care activities then nursing care is 'partly compensatory'. A further level of nursing care is educative-developmental and occurs where there are informational, motivational barriers, etc. to self-care.

Using Orem's nursing model, assessment is concerned with the identification of health deviation self-care needs, together with any universal self-care deficits. Any deficits identified are further assessed to ascertain the reason for the inability of the individual to meet self-care demands. This might be due to lack of knowledge, skill or motivation, the developmental stage, or past experience. The assessment should also identify whether or not it is safe to allow self-care.

Goals of care should be set in order of priority and formulated in discussion with the patient/client and/or family. The overriding goal is that the patient should return to full self-care activities as soon as and as far as possible.

The care plan implementation can involve informal carers and is seen as incorporating the following caring dimensions:

- Doing or acting for another
- Guiding or directing another
- Providing physical support
- Providing psychological support
- Providing an environment which supports development
- Teaching

Evaluation of care focuses upon the patient/client behaviour. That is, how far have full self-care activities been achieved?

In many ways the virtues of this model contrast with those of the Roper, Logan and Tierney model discussed above. The use of language which is very different from that to which most nurses are accustomed forces a radically different way of thinking about nursing. It is a model which is particularly useful in placing emphasis upon the patient's own role and that of the family and friends. The emphasis on patient behaviour rather than nursing actions is good, since it shifts us into identifying outcomes of care rather than concentrating upon nursing interventions.

In spite of the strange language of the model, it explicitly encourages sharing the goals of care with the patient/ client. It is a model which is particularly valuable during rehabilitation. Above all, the model can be used for health promotion activities. It fits well with the current emphasis upon individual behaviour and individual responsibility in the maintenance and promotion of health.

ORGANIZATION OF NURSING CARE IN THE WARD

When a patient goes into hospital he is asked to report to a ward which has an individual name or number. Each ward has accommodation for a number of patients ranging from around 10 in a small general hospital to as many as 40 in some general hospitals. The most usual number of beds in a ward of a general hospital is from 20 to 30. Patients are usually allocated to wards according to the specialty of the consultant. The consultant may have been allotted beds on the basis of the age of patients, the type of treatment they will undergo, or their disease. Commonly, there are adult medical, adult surgical, paediatric and elderly care wards. In larger hospitals, adult wards may be quite specialized; examples are those specializing in the care of patients with gastrointestinal complaints, neurological disease or endocrine disorders. There are usually wards reserved for the patients of the ophthalmologist and the ear, nose and throat specialist.

Trained nurses and health care assistants are employed to work upon a particular ward, whilst nurses in training progress through a planned programme of different types of nursing experience. They are allocated to a ward for experience for a period ranging from 4 to 12 weeks. The head of the nursing staff within a ward is the ward sister or charge nurse, who is responsible both to the consultants and to the Director of Nursing Services for the organization of patient care, which necessarily includes the management of the ward staff.

Task assignment

In the UK, ward nursing was traditionally organized by a system known as task assignment. Task assignment meant that for each shift, the sister or charge nurse assigned each nurse to carry out a specific nursing task for all those patients who needed it. The sister or charge nurse mentally ran through the list of patients, deciding who required a bed bath, who an 'up' bath, how many people needed mouth care, who must be routinely observed, and so on. There was also a ward routine which dictated the timetable by which these tasks were carried out.

This method of organization had the following advantages.

1. It ensured that a basic minimum of nursing care was received by each patient.
2. It allowed the use of untrained or partially trained staff, since the tasks allocated to a person could be appropriate to their skill and experience. Individuals also developed a specific skill to a high level through repeated practice.
3. It ensured that the control of patient care remained firmly in the hands of the ward sister or charge nurse as each member of staff only knew about a patient in

relation to the job they had carried out. Only the sister or charge nurse knew the full picture in respect of each patient.

4. This system allowed nurses to avoid the emotional strain of developing a close relationship with an ill patient (Menzies, 1961). Indeed, on the whole, nurses could avoid communicating with a patient altogether, except on the most superficial level.

5. Task assignment ensured that nurses did not compete for scarce equipment and facilities in the ward. For example, if only one nurse was responsible for 'up' baths, she would automatically schedule the baths so that no two patients attempted to use the bathroom at the same time as each other.

Task assignment had the following disadvantages.

1. Some of the nursing needs of a patient might fail to be recognized and so remain unfulfilled as they were not recognized as 'tasks'. Common areas of nursing needs which got neglected in task allocation were the patient's need for information, for non-directive counselling and patient teaching.

2. Care carried out as a routine of tasks might fail to fulfil the precise needs of a patient in terms of frequency, because it was aimed at the average patient. As a consequence, care might be given more frequently than needed by some patients whilst others failed to get the care they needed frequently enough. Several research studies have documented as a side issue the way in which routine care failed to meet patient need, i.e. preoperative fasting (Hamilton-Smith, 1972), bowel care (Wright, 1974), administration of postoperative analgesics (Hayward, 1975), and in general (Lelean, 1973).

3. This method of care organization was less than ideal

for nurse training. Students could not learn to assess patients' needs or to identify patients' problems. They failed to learn how to plan nursing care. Communication between student nurses and patients became difficult, since students rarely had enough information to feel free to talk with patients. They felt they were 'nursing in the dark' (Melia, 1982). When nurses were asked questions by the patient, they often did not know the answers, they did not know if they were allowed to answer and felt unsure how much the patient already knew.

4. Patients were also more likely to become dissatisfied with the care they received since they never got to know the staff members well. Neither was communication adequate between the patients and the student nurses who carried out the bulk of their care.

Team nursing

Team nursing is very similar to task assignment as a method of ward organization. Here, groups of patients, numerically smaller than the total number in the ward, and whose beds are geographically near to one another, are cared for by a team of nurses who are a subgroup of the total ward staff. For example, a modern ward may be divided into two ten-bedded rooms, a four-bedded room, and two single rooms. The staff may be divided into three teams, two caring for patients in each of the ten-bedded rooms, whilst the third team cares for the patients in the four-bedded ward and the single rooms. Within each team, one person is assigned as leader and task assignment occurs. However, because of the smaller number of patients and their greater geographical compactness, members of the team get to know the patients better and care can be more individually planned and carried out.

Patient assignment

In patient assignment, each nurse is allocated a group of patients for whose nursing care she is responsible. It will be noted that this is the method of organization in the community where a health visitor will have a caseload of 'her' clients and a district nurse will be responsible for a number of patients who need nursing care. Community nurses are usually attached to a general practice and the caseload is a function of the doctor's list. In a ward the patient's level of dependency can be carefully matched to the nurse's level of training and competence.

Advantages of patient assignment include the following.

1. Patient needs can be identified and care planned on an individual basis to meet a patient's needs.
2. A relationship can develop between nurse and patient which allows for closer emotional support, communication and the development of mutual trust. Relatives also get to know and to be known by the nurse. They can also be given information and teaching so that there will be better continuity of care between hospital and home.
3. Students gradually learn to care for patients of increasing dependency who demand more and more advanced nursing skills. Nurses use a range of different skills during any one shift, preventing boredom.
4. Nurse satisfaction is greater since each nurse is given responsibility.
5. Student nurses get to know a great deal more about their patient. They are able to communicate with him and avoid the stress of 'nursing in the dark' (Melia, 1982).

The disadvantages of patient assignment include the following.

1. Obviously patients are rarely in hospital unless they require care over a 24-hour period. It is impossible, therefore, to assign the same nurse to care for the patient the whole time. Any one nurse will work only one shift in 24 hours and will have one or more days off during a week. Inevitably then there will be changes of nurses involved in the patient's care.

2. If for some reason nurse and patient do not 'get on' with one another, they are brought into much closer contact than would be the case with task assignment.

3. The emotional challenge on the nurse is much greater with patient assignment.

4. Scarce equipment or accommodation may cause problems if more than one nurse wishes to use it at the same time.

5. The sister or charge nurse has to accept the fact that she or he may know less about an individual patient than the student nurse who is caring for him. This leads to a feeling of 'loss of control' over events in the ward and demands a good deal of adjustment to a new role.

Primary nursing

Some of the problems of coping with nurses' off-duty times mentioned in relation to patient assignment can be prevented by the use of 'primary nursing'. Primary nursing is a method of overcoming the organizational problem. In primary nursing, each nurse has a number of patients for whom she is responsible. The primary nurse interviews the patient to obtain the history, records the nursing assessment and writes the care plan. When she is away from the ward, she hands over to another nurse who gives nursing care according to the care plan until the primary nurse returns. It is the primary nurse who is responsible and accountable for the patient throughout his stay in hospital, thus ensuring continuity of care. Other nurses who help in the patient care are called 'associates'.

Several units throughout the UK organize care in this way. It is frequently associated with so-called 'nursing beds' or the 'nursing development unit', where patients are admitted to hospital specifically for nursing care on the authority of a nurse.

THE NURSING PROCESS

The nursing process consists of a description of the actions involved in nursing; it was first used in the USA. It is now used generally throughout the UK. The (1988) nursing regrading exercise used the nursing process terminology as part of the definition of many of the nursing grades.

The term describes the stages taken in carrying out nursing care. In making the stages explicit and naming them, nurses are able to evaluate what they do in terms of actions but also become aware of the mental processes involved. The object in introducing the nursing process is to improve patient care. Improved documentation also results.

Usually the nursing process is associated with patient assignment or team nursing but at least in theory it could be used with a task assignment method of ward organization.

Using a particular nursing model, stages in the nursing process comprise:

1. Collecting information about the patient:
   (a) By taking a nursing history.
   (b) By assessing the patient's condition.
   (c) By using documentary sources of information.

2. Using the information which has been collected and, through a process of inference, identifying and stating nursing problems; related nursing objectives are also identified.
3. The writing of a nursing care plan.
4. The giving of the planned nursing care.
5. The assessing of the effectiveness of care.

The whole becomes a cyclical process since further nursing problems are identified throughout the patient's stay in hospital and evaluation of care implies the reassessment of the patient (see Figure 4.1).

Collecting information about the patient

Information may be collected from primary sources, for example by asking the patient or by direct observation of the patient. It is also possible to obtain information from secondary sources, for example by asking relatives, by copying details from the admission notes or by asking the doctor the result of the examination.

The nursing history

This involves interacting with the patient and asking for information relevant to his nursing care. It can be done over the first 24 hours after admission to the care of the

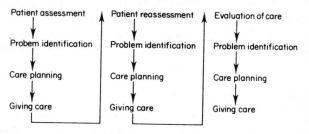

Figure 4.1 Stages of the nursing process.

nursing team so that the patient does not become over-burdened. In sitting and talking with the patient, a relationship is established which lays a firm foundation for the patient's care. Giving the nurse information reassures the patient that the staff understand his unique situation.

Usually there will be a history/assessment form available for nurses to use and this should be completed. History/assessment forms often focus upon activities of daily living so that information is collected about the patient's normal activity level, mobility, eating and drinking habits, time of sleeping, waking, etc. Impressions of any previous hospital admission and how the patient feels about the present illness may be explored. In the case of unconscious patients or young children, such information may be collected from relatives.

Nursing assessment

The assessment is carried out by observation and will include items related to the appearance of the patient's skin, posture, build, how well nourished he appears, any skin abrasions, the state of the mouth, and so on. A record will be obtained of temperature, pulse, respiration and blood pressure on admission. Some of the relevant data may be obtained from the doctor who will carry out a full physical examination of the patient.

The history and assessment are used to identify a patient's nursing problems which are the concern of the nursing staff. Many of these problems can be directly identified and stated by the patient himself but others result from the nurse's professional knowledge.

Classifying patient problems

There are several ways of classifying patients' nursing problems (Tables 4.1–4.3). One way is to classify problems as usual or unusual.

Table 4.1 An example of a nursing problem set alongside an example of a medical problem.

Nursing problem	Medical problem
Patient has difficulty in breathing unless he is sitting upright	Patient has congestive heart failure
Patient has difficulty in eating large amounts of food, and so needs small, frequent meals	

Table 4.2 Examples of usual and unusual problems.

Usual problems
   A need for information on admission
   Vomiting during an anaesthetic unless the stomach is empty
   Pain in rheumatoid arthritis

Unusual problems
   The patient had a very unpleasant experience of an anaesthetic as a
      child and is terrified of a further anaesthetic
   The patient is a vegetarian
   The patient is immobile and incontinent of urine

Table 4.3 Examples of other types of problems.

Actual problem
   The patient is dehydrated
   The patient has a foul-smelling and dry mouth

Potential problem
   The patient has to sit upright and his position can be altered very
      little, therefore there is a great risk of the development of a
      pressure sore
   The patient has had a lumbar puncture, therefore there is a risk that
      he will develop a headache

Possible problem
   During operation the patient's blood pressure was low, therefore he
      could develop kidney failure and his urinary output should be
      monitored carefully

Usual problems are those which nursing knowledge tells us are either invariable or extremely common in certain diseases or accompanying common forms of treatment. We therefore plan nursing care to prevent such problems, or to identify them and to deal with them very rapidly. *Unusual* problems are problems which are unique to the patient or otherwise uncommon.

There are other ways of classifying problems, such as: (1) *actual* problems, which are problems the patient has here and now; (2) *potential* problems, which are problems that will present unless preventive measures are taken: (3) *possible* problems, which are unlikely but should be borne in mind if certain signs and symptoms appear.

The system used to classify problems should be chosen according to its usefulness in ensuring that all a patient's existing and potential problems are identified. One of the most important ways of looking at patient problems, however, is to establish their priority so that urgent problems are dealt with first. Bower (1977) determined a hierarchy of importance in dealing with problems.

1. Problems which threaten life, the dignity and integrity of the individual, the family or the community.
2. Problems which threaten destructively to change the individual, the family or the community.
3. Problems that affect the normal developmental growth of the individual, family or community.

One could also place priority on the problems of an individual patient in the following way.

1. Problems that threaten life.
2. Problems of pain or discomfort of the patient.
3. Problems of distress of the patient.
4. Problems which might eventually lead to a threat to the patient's life.

5. Problems likely to lead to pain or discomfort.
6. Problems likely to lead to distress.
7. Problems which may complicate recovery and therefore delay it.
8. Problems which might prevent the patient from achieving realistic psychological, economic and social goals in the future.

Care planning

A plan is a hierarchical method of controlling the order in which a sequence of operations is to be performed. Patient care planning is the systematic assessment and identification of patient problems, the setting of objectives and the establishment of methods and strategies for accomplishing them (Mayers, 1978). A care plan should be a written record of identified nursing problems and the nursing actions to be taken to meet the patient's needs, including the method of evaluating the effectiveness of nursing actions. An example of a nursing care plan is shown in Figure 4.2.

Methods of giving nursing care comprise the subject matter of most of this book. Giving nursing care is an essential part of the nursing process but it may not be carried out by the person who has written the care plan. Traditionally, this is the part of the nursing process which has been given enormous emphasis in the past to the detriment of the other stages described here. Currently, there is greater emphasis on identifying the care which is appropriate, as well as on how to carry out the nursing procedures.

Evaluation of care (or reassessment)

The evaluation of the effectiveness of care should be specified in the care plan. Objectives of care may have

Figure 4.2 An example of part of a nursing care plan.

Date identified	Problem	Objective	Date begun	Nursing action	Discontinued	Evaluation
16.8.81	Dry lips, coated tongue	Lips and tongue should be moist and pink	16.8.81	Mouth care 2-hourly; to have 3000 ml of fluid daily: 1500 ml from 0800–1600; 1000 ml from 1600–2200; 500 ml from 2200–0800	21.8.81	Mouth fresh, lips and tongue moist and pink
16.8.81	Patient obese and immobile; may develop pressure sores; perspiring a lot	Healthy dry, intact skin	16.8.81	Change position every 2 hours; change sheets and wash skin 2-hourly if necessary; adjust bed clothing so that patient feels comfortably cool	21.8.81	Skin dry and intact; no redness; no numbness

been written in a form which means that achievement of the objective is itself an evaluation of effectiveness of care.

Advantages of the nursing process

Many of the advantages of using the nursing process are those of implementing patient assignment. In addition, the nursing process ensures a more complete record of the patient's condition throughout his stay, through the use of a nursing history and assessment form. Using a nursing care plan means that there is an extremely detailed record of the nursing care which the patient has received. Communication about the patient between members of staff on different shifts is more effective. The documentation allows the person in charge of the ward to monitor the patient's condition and care, and so this overcomes the feeling of loss of control experienced by the ward sister or charge nurse when patient assignment is used.

In using the nursing process there tends to be a greater emphasis on a patient's social and psychological needs and the patient can be included in the process of identifying nursing problems and the goals of care. He can then take a more active role in his own care and this prepares him more adequately for rehabilitation and discharge. Evaluating the effectiveness of care allows the matching of care to meet the patient's needs and it also can lead to constant improvement of nursing methods in the ward. Nurses learn to be more self-critical. The use of the nursing process is a good aid to student learning and in particular helps the linking of theory with practice.

5 The physical environment for care

There is an increasing awareness of factors in our environment that place our health at risk. Such factors include radioactivity from natural or artificial sources, air pollution by smoke, noxious gases from industrial processes, vehicle exhaust fumes, and water pollution. Within the work environment it is the Health and Safety Executive which has a role in securing a healthy work place. As nurses, we need to understand dangers to health which occur within the everyday environment and the means by which people's attention may be drawn to these dangers. We also need to understand the work of the Health and Safety Executive.

However, this chapter will concentrate upon the physical environment for patients and, in particular, the physical environment for hospital patients. Individuals who are ill are likely to be far more vulnerable to harm within their immediate environment than are individuals in full health. It is also the case that children and elderly people are less able than healthy young adults to resist environmental dangers.

Evolutionary processes have ensured that species that have survived environmental pressures are those able to protect themselves. Human beings are arguably the most well-adapted species and accordingly have many protective mechanisms to help survival. These mechanisms are poorly developed in infants, who depend upon their parents to protect them. In elderly people such protective mechanisms may become less efficient. In evolutionary terms, elderly people are not concerned in the survival of the species and so efficient protection beyond child-bearing age has probably not been subject to natural selection.

Table 5.1 shows some of the environmental dangers to which the human species has been exposed, together with the protective mechanisms which have evolved. Overall, man's intelligence has enabled the mastery of environmental danger.

Many of the health problems of today could be said to arise from the nature of the man-made world, at least within developed countries, and the damage which man has done to the natural world. For example, there appears to be a threat of environmental temperature change due to the damage done to the ozone layer. Another example is that, through poorly controlled use of antibiotics, pathogenic microorganisms have developed resistance to antibiotics, making infection much more difficult to treat.

Whilst microorganisms have always been present within our environment, they are also living creatures and capable of adaptation. Thus, 'new' pathogenic organisms constantly arise (that is, ones against which man has not developed specific resistance). Current examples of such organisms are the hepatitis B virus and the human immunodeficiency virus (HIV).

PATIENTS AND THE PHYSICAL ENVIRONMENT

Ill people become more vulnerable to environmental danger for several possible reasons. For example, any illness associated with vision or hearing effects or physical weakness may prevent patients from moving rapidly in the event of fire. Some patients may have poor nutritional levels due to illness, thus reducing their ability to resist

Table 5.1 Examples of environmental dangers and protective mechanisms which have evolved.

Environmental danger	Defence mechanisms
1. Trauma	Blood clotting
	Wound contraction and
	Temporary sealing
	Healing process
2. Predators	Ability to run away
3. Infection by contact	Intact skin
	Intact mucous membranes
	Antibodies
	White blood cells
	Mast cells
	Inflammatory response
4. Air-borne infection	Ciliated mucous membrane in respiratory tract
	Lymph nodes
	Coughing
5. Food-borne infection	Antiseptic property of saliva
	Hydrochloric acid in stomach
	Vomiting reflex
6. Food-borne chemical poisoning	Diarrhoea
	Vomiting
7. Burns and scalds	Withdrawal response to pain and heat
	Blood pressure and fluid homeostasis
	Healing, etc.
8. Extreme environmental temperatures	Temperature homeostasis
	Sweating
	Shivering
	Ability to put on warmer clothing, make shelter, etc.
9. Starvation	Fat stores

Note. Homeostasis and the stress response are implicated in many of the examples given.

infection. Drugs used in the treatment of disease may produce side-effects in some individuals, causing a depression in the production of white blood cells. This clearly renders the individual vulnerable to infection. The stress response can also depress resistance to infection. Invasive procedures, such as injection, catheterization, the introduction of intravenous lines and surgical operations, open up direct routes for organisms to enter the body. Unconscious patients lose many of the natural protective reflexes and this makes them more vulnerable to such complications as chest infections, urinary infections, etc. Prolonged pressure on the skin from immobility leaves the skin vulnerable to splitting and blistering, again allowing the entry of microorganisms.

THE HOSPITAL ENVIRONMENT

During a stay in hospital the ward is the patient's home, it is the place in which, confined to bed, he must spend the day, eat and sleep, and where personal toilet needs must be met. The planning of ward units has received a great deal of attention recently as new hospitals are built and older ones are modernized. Not so very many years ago the majority of patients spent most of their time in hospital in bed and were allowed to be up only for short periods at certain times of the day when convalescent. Now many patients are encouraged to get up to go to the bath and to the toilet and often spend a considerable part of the day out of bed. One feature of the newer ward units is the provision of more washing and toilet facilities and of a sitting-and-dining room where ambulant patients can have their meals, and where such recreations as playing card games and listening to radio and television can be allowed without disturbing ill patients.

The ward should be both comfortable and attractive. It

should be light and airy, kept at a comfortable temperature, and in a good decorative state. Walls and cupboards
should be decorated in washable paint or wall covering,
so that they may be cleaned regularly.

The reduction of unnecessary noise should be the aim
of every hospital and something which the nurse must
always have in mind. This depends very much on the
effort made by each individual member of the staff, but
the provision of equipment which can be handled without
noisy clatter (e.g. plastic rather than metal bins and pails) is
a great help. Moreover, in the planning of new buildings
the type of construction has a bearing on noise, and the
provision of central departments for the cleaning and
sterilization of equipment and for washing up dishes makes
the ward a much quieter place than it can possibly be
when these procedures are carried out in ward preparation
rooms and ward kitchens.

The nurse should bear in mind the need of each patient
for space and privacy. Little or no research has been
done on the psychological effects on patients of the beds
being close together, although it has long been accepted
that overcrowding of wards makes cross-infection difficult
to control. It is known that overcrowding does have
adverse behavioural effects on experimental animals. It is
not the nurse's fault, of course, if extra beds are put into
a ward in emergencies, but additional care must be taken
to ensure privacy for patients when space is cramped.
Research has shown that patients do, on the whole, prefer
to be with others in wards of around 12 to 16 beds, but
this might well be because few have the opportunity to
try single rooms. The nurse must be meticulous in drawing
curtains around the bed when intimate and personal procedures are carried out.

It has long been the case that the freedom for patients
and visitors to smoke has been curtailed within hospital

wards. Nowadays most hospitals have a non-smoking policy and visitors have to extinguish cigarettes, cigars and pipes before entering the hospital building. Unfortunately it is impossible for some patients who are highly dependent upon smoking to give it up. In such cases limited smoking may be allowed in one day room, shared by more than one ward, so leaving other day rooms for non-smokers. Clearly patients should be encouraged to stop smoking on health grounds but if this is not possible then they should be asked to confine their smoking to the day room where it is allowed.

Nursing control over the patient's environment

There are several problems associated with the ward environment for patients unfortunate enough to be admitted to hospital. Some of these have already been mentioned. They include lack of privacy, and possible overcrowding. A further problem is that of sharing the environment with others who have competing needs and tastes. For example, one patient may prefer fresh air, whilst another wishes to avoid draughts; one likes a very warm environment, another likes a cool one; one person likes absolute quiet, whilst another likes some noise. Examples of this kind are numerous.

Partly because of these competing needs, in practice it is the nursing staff who control the patient's environment, and not just in a physical sense but also in terms of the routine of daily living and in terms of the psychological atmosphere. For independent adults, having one's environment controlled by others may be extremely stressful. Any such stress will be additional to the stress of illness. It can be alleviated by allowing patients as much control over their environment as possible and by giving as much choice as possible. When this is not feasible, patients can be helped to perceive that they have some control by giving them as much information as possible about the sequence of events, the reasons why things are done, and how events will seem from the patients' point of view.

A potential source of conflict is that, to a patient, the ward is a temporary home, whilst to a member of staff it is a place of work. Staff who see the ward only as a work place may be extremely insensitive to the needs of patients.

WARD CLEANING AND MAINTENANCE

The daily cleaning of the ward and its annexes is carried out by a separate domestic staff. Dust is liable to be heavily contaminated by pathogenic organisms, so cleaning must never be carried out by those responsible for patient care. None the less, the nurse is concerned with the whole environment of the patient, and should ensure that it is clean, and that cross-infection does not occur. Nursing staff have a monitoring role in relation to the hygiene standards achieved by domestic staff. If the standards are unsatisfactory, the manager responsible for monitoring the domestic contract must be informed so that the work can be put right.

Where nursing staff are able to influence the supplies department, they should ensure that items of furniture and equipment are bought which can be washed and dried, or can be disposed of after use. Articles should have a smooth surface, with no indentations in which dirt can accumulate. Floors should be sealed with poly-urethane, or made of tiles, which can be washed. All members of the nursing staff should know the times at which routine cleaning is carried out so that they may plan dressings and other sterile procedures accordingly.

Washing bowls and baths are particularly difficult to

keep clean from the organizational point of view, since they must be cleaned between use, but there may not be a domestic worker available for this job when baths and washes are being carried out. Ideally there should be enough washing bowls for all patients, but as far as baths are concerned there is, inevitably, a shortage of these in our hospital wards. If the nurse is helping the patient with his bath, she can get the bath cleaned, but quite often up patients go to have baths at what are convenient moments for them, but finding the bath dirty, do not know how to set about getting it cleaned, and do not like to worry busy people. There is no reason why cleaning materials cannot be left available so that patients can clean the bath after use, as they would at home. Otherwise, they must be told to ask the domestic worker to clean it for them.

Beds and lockers should be thoroughly washed over with an antiseptic solution and dried when a patient has been discharged. Clean bed linen, blankets and pillows will be used to make up the bed when it has been washed.

Clean linen is usually brought to the ward each day to maintain a constant supply of each article in the linen cupboard. Dirty linen is put into bags and these are collected by the laundry porter. Nursing staff are responsible for keeping dirty linen from infectious patients separate from other linen. For certain diseases, specific policies will be in force for the safe disposal of linen. These policies must be followed.

The ward kitchen

In general, the cleanliness of the ward kitchen is the responsibility of domestic staff. Nursing staff should ensure that any spilled food or milk is cleaned up immediately, for fear of accidents.

Refrigerators should be defrosted and washed thoroughly by the domestic staff at regular intervals, at least once a week, and more frequently during hot weather. Surplus food supplied to the ward should be returned to the kitchen for disposal.

Bedpans and urinals

Bedpans and urinals are the concern of the nursing staff. They should be flushed with cold water after use, then rinsed with disinfectant. Next, automatic bedpan washers in which the bedpan can be enclosed to be flushed with cold and hot water should be used, and finally when it is clean, it should be sterilized in a tank of boiling water. (Minimum time for immersion in boiling water is 5 min.) It is essential that the bedpan is cleaned of all organic matter before being put in the sterilizer because organic matter provides a protective covering for microorganisms, which thus escape destruction during the boiling process. However, the use of disposable bedpans is the method of choice.

CROSS-INFECTION

One danger to which a patient is exposed when in hospital to a far greater extent than at home is cross-infection. Cross-infection can be defined as the transmission of infection from one person to another, or from one site on an individual to another site on the *same* person.

Nosocomial infection is infection acquired by a patient through the medium of a member of staff, e.g. from the hands of staff or equipment they are using.

Factors associated with hospitals which contribute to the potential danger of infection are:

1. The high degree of patient contact with strangers,

such as other patients, the relatives and friends of other patients, doctors, nurses, therapists, porters, medical students, auxillary workers, chaplains, etc.

2. People who make contact with patients in hospital, particularly the staff, may be carrying organisms which are pathogenic (i.e. disease producing). Further, there is a real danger that such pathogenic organisms have developed resistance to antibiotics. Hospital staff are far more likely to carry pathogenic and antibiotic-resistant pathogenic organisms than are members of the general public.

3. Patients are probably more vulnerable to infection than healthy people. This might be due to the side-effects of drugs, the type of illness (e.g. leukaemia) or to raised stress levels, which can result in lowered levels of circulating neutrophils and/or suppression of the inflammatory response.

4. Patients are also more vulnerable to infection as a result of wounds or invasive procedures which provide direct entry of organisms into the body, bypassing the protection of intact skin or mucous membranes.

Hepatitis B and HIV precautions

In recent years additional precautions have become necessary to protect both patients and staff from the possibility of becoming infected with the hepatitis B virus or the human immunodeficiency virus (HIV). The risk from hepatitis B is much greater than from HIV because the latter is a fragile virus which cannot survive well outside human body fluid. Precautions taken to prevent hepatitis B infection are more than adequate to prevent HIV infection. Both viruses are potentially dangerous in relation to needle stick injuries open skin lesions and blood products.

Needle stick injuries

Here, the danger is from injury with needles which have been used in the treatment of a patient who is infected. We now have some clear guidelines to prevent such injuries:

1. Needles should never be replaced into the sheath after use for hypodermic, intramuscular or intravenous injections.
2. Instead they should be placed into a special container for disposable sharps. Such containers should be robust, so that needles cannot poke through the sides, and must never be overfilled.

Treatment and preparation rooms

In modern hospital wards, provision is made for dressings and other sterile procedures to be carried out in a treatment room, away from the ward. Adjacent to the treatment room are two annexes, one a 'clean' preparation room where sterile equipment and lotions are stored and trolleys can be laid. The other annexe is a 'dirty' utility room where instruments are washed and boiled, ready for return to the central sterile supply department. Dirty dressings will have been placed straight into a paper bag during the dressing. The bag should now be closed gently, taking care not to cause a great upward puff of air from the bag in the process, and sealed with tape before being put into the polythene-lined dirty dressing bin. Used disposables should be put into a separate polythene-lined bin. These bins are emptied by a special porter.

Ideally, the treatment room will be air-conditioned, but in many modernized wards rooms have been adapted as treatment rooms, rather than being purpose built, and an air-conditioning system is not possible. Every possible precaution should be taken to keep both the treatment and the 'clean' preparation room as dust free as possible. All surfaces must be washable, equipment should be placed in closed cupboards, windows should be closed, and no one should be allowed into the rooms unnecessarily.

If dressings have to be carried out in the ward then it is especially important that the number of organisms in the air is kept to a minimum because they can be breathed in or get on to surfaces and bedclothes. Activities in the ward such as bed making should disturb the air as little as possible. Surfaces should be cleaned in a way that will prevent dust from rising in the air, thus vacuum cleaning and washing of floors, rather than sweeping, and washing surfaces with an antiseptic instead of dusting, is advocated.

So that a nurse may maintain the best physical environment for her patients, in which there is no danger to them from cross-infection, she should understand the principles of microbiology, the conditions under which microorganisms survive and multiply, and the ways in which their growth may be inhibited. Given this understanding, her nursing techniques will be safe and she will be capable of advising and supervising the domestic staff in the cleaning of the ward.

Microorganisms

Microorganisms, for the most part, are either positively helpful to man (soil organisms are an example), or at least do no harm. Some, however, are capable of causing diseases, and it is these with which the doctors and nurses are concerned. Harmful (pathogenic) organisms need fairly well-defined environmental conditions for their growth.

The word 'growth', when used of microorganisms, refers not to the organisms getting physically bigger, as a human does, but to the multiplication of the unicellular organism, by cellular division, to form many identical microorganisms. Under ideal conditions a microorganism may divide at 20-minute intervals. Thus, one cell divides to form two, then these in turn divide, forming four in all, and so on. It can be seen that it is most important to prevent this happening.

Their requirements for multiplication include a narrow range of temperature (around human body temperature), and of acidity—alkalinity. They also need both moisture and food substances in their environment. Thus the multiplication of many pathogenic organisms can be inhibited by depriving them of moisture; this is why surfaces should be dried and kept dry. Very high, or very low temperatures, will inhibit their growth, and a temperature of 100°C (212°F) for 5 minutes will actually kill most pathogenic organisms. Some chemicals, the disinfectants and antiseptics, cause damage to the cellular components of the organism, whilst antibiotics interfere with their metabolism. Gamma radiation destroys microorganisms and is an excellent method of sterilization for prepacked dressings and equipment.

Some microorganisms have the capacity to protect themselves from adverse conditions, only to begin multiplying when conditions again suit their requirements. These organisms are termed 'spore-forming' organisms, and they are more difficult to kill than non-spore-forming organisms. For instance, boiling for 5 minutes will not kill them, but higher temperatures, as produced by steam under pressure, will.

STERILIZATION

Sterilization in the microbiological sense means the process whereby a substance or body is rendered free from living organisms, and under this term are included various methods of killing bacteria and other microorganisms.

All instruments, utensils and dressings used in the conduct of surgical dressings and other procedures for which aseptic precautions are necessary must be sterile and must then be handled only by a person with sterilized gloved hands or with sterile forceps.

The word 'asepsis' implies the absence of microorganisms, while 'antisepsis' (against sepsis) usually implies the use of chemical disinfectants to kill microorganisms. Aseptic precautions in a ward or theatre imply that all dressings and appliances are sterile and that there is no risk of contaminating the wound. While similar precautions are taken with septic cases, additional antiseptic precautions may be taken to prevent spread of infection.

It cannot be too strongly emphasized that all dressing utensils and materials must be kept free from contamination with gross dirt, even if they are to be sterilized before use. Any method of sterilization will be ineffective unless the equipment is thoroughly cleaned beforehand. Any organic matter, such as blood, pus or excreta, will form a barrier to full penetration by the sterilizing agent. A further point which is not always appreciated is that aseptic precautions are as necessary in dealing with an infected wound as with a clean one. The danger to the patient is increased if a fresh infection is introduced.

Sterilization of instruments and equipment used in surgical practice is usually effected by exposure to high temperatures for a sufficient length of time to kill all living organisms, including spore-forming organisms.

Other physical means such as exposure to gamma rays in an atomic pile or irradiation by radioactive cobalt are used and are particularly useful for sterilizing equipment which is readily damaged by heat, such as rubber articles and some endoscopes. Within the hospital, however, heat is the most generally used, and the most efficient agent, wherever its use is possible, in the form of high-pressure steam sterilizers (autoclaves) and hot-air ovens.

Disinfection by chemical agents is an ancillary method for materials and equipment which cannot stand exposure to heat, such as some endoscopes; chemical agents are also used for disinfection of the skin and the irrigation of body cavities.

Sterilization by physical means

Sufficient heat over a sufficiently long period of time kills all forms of bacterial life, although those organisms which can take on a protective spore formation can withstand a higher temperature for a longer period than the less resistant, or vegetative, forms.

Autoclaving

Steam kills organisms by coagulation of the cell protein, provided that certain factors are present; the steam must be under pressure, dry and saturated. With these conditions fulfilled, the steam will condense when it meets the cooler surface of the articles in the autoclave, and the latent heat released on condensation will penetrate and kill the organisms. Autoclaving at a pressure of 220 kPa (20 lb/in^2) (above atmospheric pressure) and a temperature of 126°C (260°F) for 20 minutes is an efficient method of sterilizing fabrics such as gowns, towels and dressings, and also instruments. The latest types of high-speed, high-vacuum autoclave operating at higher temperatures reduce the time needed for sterilization. Prepacked dressings supplied to wards have usually been sterilized by the method outlined above. Before use, dates and sterilization strips should be checked.

It is important to remember that any sterilization by autoclaving is reliable only if the autoclave is correctly installed and efficiently operated, and the materials are packed loosely so that all parts are accessible to the steam. The operation of an autoclave is a serious responsibility and should be entrusted only to one who understands its working. Tests of efficiency, in addition to checking the accuracy of the pressure gauges and temperature readings, should be carried out at regular intervals; these include indicators, control tubes and bacteriological tests.

Dry heat

Dry heat kills microorganisms by oxidation, and provided that the articles to be sterilized are exposed to a temperature of 160°C (320°F) for 1 hour, all organisms and their spores will be destroyed. This method is suitable for all types of glassware, including all glass syringes (but not glass and metal syringes where solder will melt in the high temperature in the oven) and some instruments such as knife blades and skin-grafting knives.

Other physical agents

Other physical agents in addition to heat will destroy bacteria, but, with the exception of gamma radiation, have not a very wide practical application in hospital practice.

Cold. Most organisms will survive exposure to very low temperatures but will not multiply. A practical application of this is the preservation of foodstuffs in cold storage.

Light. Direct sunlight kills many bacteria, including *Mycobacterium tuberculosis.* The active agent is the ultra-violet radiation and these rays have been used to sterilize milk and water.

Drying. Moisture is as important to most bacterial cells as it is to tissue cells, and removal of water will kill the cell. In certain circumstances, however, some bacteria can survive drying for considerable periods and are therefore likely to be present in dust. Examples are pyogenic organisms, diphtheria bacillus and the *Mycobacterium tuberculosis* in pus and sputum.

Gamma radiation. This agent is being increasingly used for materials which cannot be effectively sterilized by heat without damage. A number of packaged disposable items of surgical equipment, such as plastic catheters, knife holders and tubing, and suture materials are also sterilized by this method.

Boiling This method may be used in an emergency, but it is not recommended.

All pathogenic organisms in the vegetative form are killed by 5-minute immersion in boiling water, but the method is particularly open to human error.

1. The water must be boiling for the full 5 minutes. The addition of cold articles takes the water off the boil and timing must begin from when the water begins to boil again.
2. All articles must be completely immersed in the boiling water.
3. Articles must be spotlessly clean before being immersed in the boiling water. Blood, pus and excreta form a barrier, protecting the organism from the boiling water.
4. For articles to remain sterile, they must be removed from the boiling water by means of sterile handling

forceps, and must be placed on to a sterile surface and covered with a sterile lid, so that complete protection from contamination is obtained.

5. A major source of danger of this method is that articles are wet when removed from the boiling water and moisture aids the growth of microorganisms. Thus the articles must not be contaminated with microorganisms.

6. The articles to be sterilized must be constructed of materials not damaged by boiling water, and should be so constructed that all surfaces are in contact with the boiling water.

Nowadays, all sterile equipment required for dressings and other procedures is sterilized centrally and delivered to the ward daily. Usually all the equipment required for a dressing or other technique is packed in a bag and then sterilized by steam under pressure. The nurse then needs to choose the appropriate pack and use an aseptic technique for the dressing. Syringes may be sterilized centrally in a hot oven, but usually disposable syringes are used. These are sterilized by the manufacturers. Many other disposables are sterilized by gamma radiation by the manufacturers and remain sterile until the packet is opened. Catheters, disposable instruments, airways and stomach tubes are common examples.

Chemical disinfectants

It is essential that the nurse should understand the necessary conditions for the effective use of these agents, otherwise chemical disinfection may be quite useless and may even be dangerous if it gives rise to a false sense of security. Therefore, dilution instructions must be followed meticulously.

1. To be efficient the disinfectant must be sufficiently strong and must be allowed to act for a sufficient length of time.

2. With very few exceptions, the disinfectant must be in solution; dry powders have very little effect.

3. The disinfecting power of the agent varies with the number of organisms present; highly infected material is difficult to disinfect efficiently.

4. The disinfecting power of the agent is to a certain extent dependent upon the nature of the medium containing the organisms, e.g. the germicidal power is lowered in the presence of pus since, in this medium, many of the organisms are inside the dead leukocytes and thus it is difficult for the disinfectant to reach them.

5. As a general rule it may be stated that disinfectant solutions are more effective hot than cold.

6. Spore-forming bacteria and the acid-fast group (of which the *Mycobacterium tuberculosis* is the most important member) are much more resistant to the action of liquid disinfectants than they are to the action of heat.

6   Admission of patients

.Whether or not a patient remains at home or is admitted to hospital when ill makes a tremendous difference to the admission process. Admission to hospital is a very significant event for a patient, with all the hidden meanings which are implied by the admission. At the very least it means separation from family and friends, and making many new adjustments. These include an entirely new routine of daily living and living for a time within a rather alien environment. It also implies the presence of an illness too serious to be treated by the doctor in the surgery or in the patient's own home (Kornfield, 1979). Perhaps it is not too surprising that much of this chapter will be concerned with the admission of the patient to hospital.

There is however a procedure to be followed by the district nurse when a patient is referred for district nursing by the practitioner or hospital. The nurse must make an initial visit to the patient's home to introduce herself. At this point the situation is very different from that of the hospital admission, since the district nurse is a guest in the patient's home and is there only by consent of the patient and not by right. The patient will dictate the pace of events. Having effected introductions, however, the qualified district nurse will go on to carry out a full nursing assessment of the patient, identifying the nursing problems using a relevant nursing model.

Goals of care are formulated and a written care plan is

developed which specifies the nursing interventions required. This plan is left in the patient's home. If relatives are to help with care then they need to be given clear instructions and help. The help of other agencies may be required, in which case the patient is informed of this before the nurse carries out the referral. Finally the nurse decides whether care is to be delegated to less highly qualified staff and the patient is informed of their names and their roles before the district nurse leaves the patient.

ADMISSION TO HOSPITAL

First impressions of a hospital may colour the subsequent experiences of that hospital for a patient, who will be feeling apprehensive about the treatment, about the lack of privacy in the ward, and about leaving family and friends. By considering the patient's feelings, the hospital staff can help in achieving quick and easy adjustment to hospital life, and give confidence in the treatment to be received. A patient's first contact with a member of the hospital staff may well be with a porter at the gate lodge or administrative block, who will direct the patient to the ward. Sometimes necessary forms are filled in by a clerk in an admissions or reception office before the patient proceeds to the ward itself. Clear direction signs and ward names will help the patient; all members of staff should be encouraged to think of themselves as engaged in public relations as they walk along hospital corridors and in the grounds. Members of staff may well be stopped and asked the way to a ward by an anxious patient, and a friendly manner together with clear instructions can be a great help.

The ward staff will always have been notified of the patient's admission, and can help to make him feel welcome by turning back the bed and putting out water, glass and towels in readiness. When a ward is very busy, the staff may all be occupied in caring for their patients, and a new patient and the relatives can wait anxiously at the ward door for some little time before being noticed. Sometimes it is the domestic assistant who is the first to greet the new patient. Good ward organization could ensure that the nurse assigned to care for this patient is available to welcome the patient the minute he appears. A friendly welcome from the nurse and an introduction will help the patient to feel at home. He can then be seated, together with the relatives, whilst the nurse obtains any information that is required immediately. If the patient and relatives have had a long, exhausting journey to reach the hospital, they can be shown where the lavatory is and offered tea and food.

When the patient is shown to the bed, he should be introduced to the patients on either side. It is usual to ask the patient to undress and get into bed, but it is worth considering whether this is absolutely necessary for a little while, or whether it is possible for the patient to sit in the day room and get accustomed to the surroundings, the other patients, and the staff, before being asked to put on, in the middle of the day, clothes usually worn at night. Of course, some people may feel happier in pyjamas and dressing gown, since then they will be less conspicuous amongst the other patients; but for others, their normal clothing will help them to feel at less of a disadvantage when dealing with the staff.

Some patients will need to get into bed straight away, because they are exhausted after the journey; because they are to be examined; or because observations and tests will begin straight away. It may be necessary for the nurse to help the patient to undress if unable to do this for himself and there is no relative who can help.

It is rare for suitable individual accommodation to be

available for the patient's clothing. A communal cupboard is often provided and, since all patients' clothing in the ward is placed in this, it is necessary that each item of clothing is carefully labelled with the patient's name before it is put away. All the patient's belongings are carefully listed in duplicate so that a record of all property within the hospital is kept by the ward and a copy given to the patient. Patients are advised not to have valuables with them; these are locked in the hospital safe after a careful record of them has been made. Many hospitals persuade the relatives to take home all but the bare essentials that the patient will need whilst in hospital. This absolves the hospital of responsibility for belongings not directly in the patient's own care.

Patients may be asked if they are willing to put on an identiband on admission. If the patient is agreeable, then this should be completed and applied to wrist or ankle.

Care of the patient's relative

Once the patient has been settled in bed, or shown the day room if allowed up, some time is given to say goodbye to the accompanying relative. Before the relative leaves the hospital, a telephone number and address should be obtained so that contact may be made in emergencies. Information about visiting hours and the hospital procedure for telephone enquiries should be explained and, if there are likely to be difficulties in visiting at the stated hours, alternative arrangements can be made. Any information about the patient's course of treatment should be given before the relative leaves, and he can be asked to bring anything further the patient needs, during visiting hours. If the patient is unable to act as an informant for any reason, a nursing history is obtained from the relative instead.

Information the patient will need

The patient will need information about the ward routine, the layout of the ward, and how to identify members of staff. So that he is not overburdened with information, this can be given a little at a time, during the admission procedure. To reduce uncertainty, information about treatment should be given as soon as it is known. The reason for everything that is done should be carefully explained, and the patient should be carefully prepared for the effect of various procedures, i.e. what they will feel like.

Persons to be notified of admission

The following persons should be told of the patient's admission.

1. The minister of the patient's particular religion.
2. The porter dealing with the patient's post, telephone queries and directing visitors.
3. The admissions office, if they do not already know.
4. The house doctor in charge of the patient.
5. The dietitian, if the patient is on a special diet.

There may well be others who should be informed as well.

OBTAINING A NURSING HISTORY AND CARRYING OUT A NURSING ASSESSMENT

When the patient has settled in the ward and has been given the information he requires, the nurse taking responsibility for this patient's care can begin to collect a nursing history. It may also be possible to carry out at least a partial nursing assessment at the same time.

The nursing history should be obtained systematically using a form designed for the purpose (Figure 6.1). it may not be necessary (or possible) to collect all the information at once. Some of the information can be collected gradually over the first 24 hours of the patient's stay, although of course the patient may continue to reveal relevant information throughout the hospital stay, provided that a good relationship is established. As with so many other nursing activities, it is worth remembering that obtaining a nursing history serves more than one purpose. It is the time when a good nurse–patient relationship can begin to be established. For this reason the nurse should sit by the patient and take time and care in interacting. Over and above this, the patient may feel reassured that someone is not only taking an interest in him but is collecting detailed and individual information to help in planning care. For a patient (or relative) it can be frightening to think that the patient is in the care of someone (doctor or nurse) who is not in full possession of the unique history, with the consequent danger of misunderstanding or misdiagnosing what has happened. Finally, in giving a history some of the patient's fears may be brought out into the open. Through a cathartic effect this may in itself help. It also allows the fears to be dealt with.

Types of information

It is not possible to specify the information which is required from every patient as this will be modified (1) by ward requirements, and (2) by the individual patient. However, there are broad categories of information which are always needed.

1. Demographic information such as the patient's name, age, next of kin, address, occupation etc.

Figure 6.1 Example of a nursing history form.

Name	Age
Home address	Date of birth
	Sex
	Marital status
	Religion
	Admission date
	Admission time
Tel. no.	

Elimination
Fluid
Disturbed at night?
Difficulties?

Elimination
Bowel
Frequency
Pain
Constipation
Special diet
Drugs

Mental state
Alertness
Orientation
Speech
Ability to communicate
Emotional state
Memory
Attitude to hospital admission

General appearance
Build
Posture
Colour
Distinctive features

Occupation
Next of kin
Relationship
Name
Address

Tel. no.

Previous hospital admission
Date
Reason
Attitude to experience

Social history
Family
Dependants
Housing
Occupation
Likely visitors

Diet
Appetite
Indigestion
Food likes
    dislikes
Special diet

Fluid
Normal intake
Likes
Dislikes
Special problems
State of hydration

Menstruation
Regularity
Next expected period date
Method of coping
    Towels   Tampons
    Use of drugs

Sleep
Normal time of going to bed
Normal time of rising
No. of hours of sleep
Normal nightcap
Drugs
Difficulty

Mobility
Full
Restricted
Needs help with walking
Needs help with movement from bed to chair
Needs help with movement in bed
Restricted for medical reasons

Hearing
Normal
Difficulty
Hearing aid

Eyesight
Normal
Difficulty
Spectacles
Contact lenses

Mouth
Dentures
State of teeth
Mouth problems

State of skin
Abrasions
Sores
Rash
Allergy
Normal colour
Oedema

Drugs
List those taken at home

Any known allergies

Breathing
Any difficulty
a) climbing stairs
b) walking
c) sitting
d) lying flat
Are respirations easy

2. Health information, including present diagnosis (if known), symptoms, past health problems, previous admissions to hospital, allergies, etc.
3. The patient's perception of the reason for admission, his view of hospital admission, whether there is anything he is worried about or fears particularly.
4. The patient's description of the usual pattern of daily living activities such as sleep, diet, activity, bowel habits, etc.

Such information should be obtained in a friendly, leisurely and interested manner to encourage the patient to be open and frank.

Whilst the history is being taken, a certain amount of assessment can also take place. The nurse can begin to observe such things as whether the patient reveals any difficulties in understanding questions through deafness or other factors or, on the other hand, if there are any problems in communication. The nurse can observe for signs of emotion and, if so, the relationship to what is being said at the time. This gives the opportunity to encourage the patient to talk further and to counsel if appropriate. The patient's posture may also be revealing of emotional state and feelings. Depression and feelings of aggression are often revealed by characteristic postures. Physical aspects of appearance may be noted: for example, colour, nutritional state, any apparent self-neglect, breathing difficulties, abnormal movements, weakness of a part of his body, any obvious skin lesions.

More formal physical assessment will depend upon the admitting nurse's judgement of what is required. Detailed assessment is justified in the case of unconscious and seriously ill patients, when it will also be necessary to collect the nursing history from relatives or a friend. For all patients, temperature, pulse, respiration and blood pressure levels will be recorded and charted on admission, as will the result of urinalysis. When information has been collected and patient problems determined, then a nursing care plan will be written (see Chapter 4).

EMERGENCY ADMISSION

For a patient who is being admitted as an emergency, the most urgent need will be for treatment of the physical condition. He will no doubt also be very apprehensive about coming into hospital, but the predominant feeling will be one of relief at being admitted in order to get expert care and attention. He may be feeling very ill, or may be in great pain. When the ward is informed that such a patient is to be admitted, it is important that as much information as possible is obtained about the condition, so that the bed can be suitably prepared, any equipment that may be required for emergency treatment can be placed in readiness at the bedside, and a preliminary nursing care plan can be written.

Preparation of bed and equipment

The bedclothes are prepared into a 'pack' so that they can be removed in one operation from the bed when the patient arrives in the ward. This means that the patient can be lifted straight from the stretcher on to the bed; the pack can then be unfolded and the bedclothes placed in position over the patient and tucked in, in the usual way. If the patient has been involved in a road traffic accident, or has been vomiting, it may be advisable to protect the bed-linen from being soiled.

Requirements

Equipment needed in preparation at the patient's bedside

will vary according to the condition, but examples are
given below.

- Bed blocks to raise the foot of the bed ⎱ if patient is
- Intravenous infusion trolley   ⎰ shocked
- Injection tray
- Anaesthetic instruments
- Denture container
- Suction apparatus with catheters ⎱ for unconscious patient
- Identification bracelet
- Oxygen and equipment
  for its administration   ⎱ for patient in respiratory failure
- Extra pillows
- Dressing trolley and shaving tray, if patient has an
  open wound.

Reception of the patient

When the patient arrives in the ward, the relative is
asked to wait, whilst the nurse supervises the lifting of
the patient from the trolley to the bed. If the patient's
condition is critical, treatment may have to be instituted
while the patient is still on the trolley. The nurse should
assess the patient's condition, taking any emergency
measures that are necessary, and should also get a message
sent to the doctor in charge that the patient has arrived,
together with information about his condition. The
patient's fears and apprehensions should not be forgotten,
but the best way to reassure is to ensure safety and
comfort as soon as possible. Explanations of all that is
being done should be given, although of course elaborate
explanations are not required by a very ill patient. Ideally,
another nurse should see the relatives and reassure them
that the patient is receiving treatment and attention. If
no relative has accompanied the patient, steps should be

taken as soon as possible to inform the next of kin of the patient's admission. After the patient's physical needs have been attended to, the admission details can be obtained, together with such nursing history details as are appropriate, and the relatives allowed to see the patient. If immediate operation is planned, a consent form will have to be signed, and preparations for the operation carried out; this latter may include aspiration of the patient's stomach if a meal has recently been eaten.

THE DOCTOR'S EXAMINATION OF THE PATIENT

The doctor will carry out a full examination of the patient once the condition of the patient permits, in the case of an emergency admission, or at a mutually convenient time for a patient admitted from the waiting list. A great deal of information about the patient's condition can be gained by the nurse who is present to look after the patient during the examination, by observing for any obvious abnormality that is revealed during the course of the examination. If the nurse shows an intelligent interest, the doctor will probably be willing to explain the patient's signs and symptoms and their significance.

Requirements

- Ophthalmoscope (to examine the optic disc)
- Auriscope (to examine the ear drum)
- Visual acuity charts
- Hat pins with coloured ends (to test visual fields and sensation to pin prick)
- Cotton wool (to test sensation of light touch and corneal reflex)
- Hot and cold water in test tubes (to test temperature sense)

- Spatula and torch (to examine tongue, throat and palatal movement)
- Patella hammer (to test tendon reflexes)
- Tuning fork (to check hearing and vibration sense)
- Tubes containing oil of cloves, peppermint, almond, salt, sugar (to test taste and smell)
- Sphygmomanometer (to record blood pressure)
- Stethoscope (to listen to heart and respiratory sounds)
- Tape measure (to check for any bony or soft tissue deformity)
- Glove and petroleum jelly (for rectal examination)

Note. In specialist wards, routine examinations include those of special organs, e.g. vagina, ear, nose, throat.

When the doctor has completed the examination, the patient should be made comfortable and the bed straightened, before the curtains are drawn back. A word from the doctor to explain any further investigations or the line of treatment will help to reassure the patient. In any case, before leaving, the nurse should ensure that the patient is comfortable, has understood any information given by the doctor, and has been given the opportunity to ask questions. Any additional information gained about the patient's condition should be recorded on the nursing history/assessment sheets and the nursing care plan modified if necessary.

PART II: Care related to daily living activities

7   Nutrition

All organisms require food and water to maintain life. Food consists of several basic components of different chemical composition, and there is a minimum amount of each of these components which must be taken in the diet to prevent deficiency disease. However, in highly developed countries there is a great diversity of foods which will fulfil the basic needs, and what an individual actually eats will depend upon cultural and individual preference as well as on the amount of pleasure the particular individual gets from eating.

COMPONENTS OF FOOD

Carbohydrates

The basic units of carbohydrates are the rather small sugar molecules, which are made of carbon, hydrogen and oxygen. Hundreds of sugar molecules may be combined to form the large molecules, starch and glycogen, whilst the molecular form in which other carbohydrates are found in the diet is that of two sugar molecules combined together. In the body, carbohydrates are split into their component simple sugar molecules and are transported in the bloodstream in this form. These substances are then oxidized by the body cells to form carbon dioxide and water, releasing some energy as heat and storing the remaining energy obtained to perform chemical or physical work. Some sugar molecules are incorporated into the body structure, but the majority contribute toward the total kilojoule (energy producing) content of food. Fruit, sugar, potatoes, flour, bread and rice are the main sources of carbohydrate. Cellulose, a large-molecule carbohydrate, cannot be split into its component parts by the enzymes contained in the human digestive juices, and thus it passes unaltered through the alimentary tract. Cellulose is contained in fruit and vegetables; it performs the useful function of stimulating peristalsis. Cellulose is one of the substances known as dietary fibre. The importance of dietary fibre is increasingly recognized (see below).

Fat

The terms 'fat' or 'lipid' refer to a variety of different types of molecules, e.g. neutral fats, sterols and phospholipids, which form constituents of cells. Dietary fat includes neutral fat molecules which, like carbohydrates, contain carbon, hydrogen and oxygen. Fat has the property of releasing more energy per unit weight than glucose. Neutral fat molecules are normally formed of glycerol with three units of fatty acid. Fatty acids may be saturated or unsaturated. Any fat taken in excess of requirements can be stored in fat depots in the body. Excess glucose is also converted into fat and stored in this form. Lipid is an important constituent of cell membranes and this is of special importance in relation to cells within the nervous system. Their membranes may be thick, highly elaborate and contain a high proportion of fat.

Fat from animal sources, such as meat, butter, eggs and milk, contain both cholesterol and high proportions of saturated fatty acids. Vegetable oils, e.g. olive oil, sunflower oil and nut oils, are characteristically liquid at room temperature and contain high proportions of unsaturated fatty acids.

Protein

Protein is the only source of nitrogen in food, and if adequate quantities of protein-containing foods are not eaten, kwashiorkor may result. Proteins are very large molecules composed of many smaller compounds, the amino acids, of which there are 20. Some of these amino acids must be obtained from the diet (the essential amino acids), whilst others can be built up by the body, given adequate quantities of protein. Amino acids contain carbon, hydrogen, oxygen and nitrogen. They are used in the body to form enzymes, protoplasm, plasma proteins and hormones. Like fat, they are also essential components of cell membranes. Any amino acid taken in the diet in excess of the requirements for replacement and growth is converted to fat or glucose and used to obtain energy. The part of the molecule containing nitrogen is converted into urea and excreted in the urine.

Meat, fish, cheese, eggs and milk are good sources of protein in which can be found all the essential amino acids. Protein from a vegetable source (peas, beans, nuts, cereals) may not contain all the essential amino acids, so a variety of different protein foods is required daily if a vegetarian diet is strictly adhered to.

Mineral salts

Small amounts of mineral salts are found in the body. Some of these help to maintain the osmotic pressure and pH of body fluids, some are structural components of bone, whilst others are combined in large organic molecules to form enzymes, coenzymes, haemoglobin, myoglobin and hormones. Mineral salts must be present in the diet to maintain health. Those required are: potassium, sodium chloride, calcium, phosphorus, magnesium, iron, copper, zinc, iodine and manganese. Iron, calcium and iodine are those most likely to be deficient in the diet. Meat, molasses, eggs, wholemeal bread and some green vegetables contain *iron*; milk and cheese contain *calcium*, and it is added to flour other than wholemeal. *Iodine* is found in fish and foods grown in iodine-containing soil (i.e. soil which is not too far distant from the sea). Table salt may have iodine added to it. *Fluorine* is found in variable amounts in drinking water and protects against dental caries in children. In large quantities, however, it causes mottling of the teeth.

Vitamins

'Vital amines' as their name implies, are essential to life, although they do not provide energy and are required only in minute quantities. Some are soluble in fat and are absorbed from the digestive tract along with fat, while others are soluble in water.

Fat-soluble vitamins

Absorption of fat-soluble vitamins may be poor in the absence of bile or pancreatic lipase.

Vitamin A is a constituent of the visual pigment retinene and is, therefore, essential for normal vision. It also maintains the epithelial tissue of the body. Foods containing vitamin A are: meat, fish, fish liver oils, butter and cheese. Carotene, found in tomatoes and carrots, is converted into vitamin A in the body. Excessive intake of vitamin A can occur, and leads to gastrointestinal disturbance, scaly dermatitis and bone pain.

Vitamin D increases absorption of calcium and phosphorus from the digestive tract and, in its absence, rickets, a disease in which calcium is removed from the bone and teeth, may occur. Vitamin D is found in milk, butter, fish and fish liver oils. It is added to margarine. It is possible to take vitamin D in excess, leading to calcification of soft tissue.

Vitamin E: there is no evidence of the effects of deficiency of this vitamin in man, but in experimental animals vitamin E deficiency has been found to cause muscular dystrophy and fetal death. It is found in milk, eggs, meat and leafy vegetables.

Vitamin K is essential for the formation in the liver of prothrombin. Prothrombin, in turn, is an essential factor in the clotting of blood. Since bile and pancreatic lipase are necessary in order to absorb vitamin K, the clotting properties of the blood should be checked before an operation on a patient who has some biliary obstruction. Vitamin K is found in most green vegetables.

Water-soluble vitamins

Vitamin B is a complex of different vitamins: thiamine, riboflavin, niacin, pyridoxine, pantothenic acid, biotin, folic acid and cyanocobalamin. These are essential components of enzymes or coenzymes concerned in intermediary metabolism. *Vitamin B_1*, or *thiamine*, is found in liver and unrefined cereals. Deficiency diseases associated with it are beriberi and neuritis. Deficiency of *riboflavin*, or *vitamin B_2*, leads to glossitis and dermatitis around the mouth, nose, vulva and scrotum. It is found in liver and milk. The *niacin* deficiency disease is pellagra. Yeast, meat and liver contain niacin. *Pyridoxine*, or *vitamin B_6*, is also found in yeast and liver, and in wheat and corn. Its deficiency leads to mental confusion, depression and dermatitis. *Pantothenic acid* is found in eggs, liver and yeast; dermatitis, enteritis, alopecia and adrenal insufficiency may occur if it is deficient in the diet. *Biotin* is thought to be synthesized by intestinal organisms. Deficiency has been produced in man by the intake of large quantities of raw egg white. The symptoms were dermatitis, anaemia and muscle pain. *Folic acid* is essential for cell formation by division; deficiency manifests itself by sprue and anaemia. It is found in leafy green vegetables. *Vitamin B$_{12}$*, or *cyanocobalamin*, is found in liver, meat, eggs and milk. Dietary deficiency is rare, but deficiency can occur due to malabsorption through the stomach wall, as in pernicious anaemia.

Vitamin C: the action of this vitamin has not been fully determined. It is concerned in the metabolism of some amino acids and it seems to be essential for the formation of collagen. It is found concentrated in endocrine glands, especially in the adrenal cortex, and depletion of ascorbic acid (vitamin C) from the adrenal gland occurs in physiological stress. Dietary deficiency of the vitamin results in scurvy, a disease in which there are subcutaneous bruises, haemorrhage from the gums, anaemia and delay in healing. Vitamin C is found in vegetables, fruit and milk, but it is very easily destroyed by heat and exposure to light.

Kilojoule requirements

Neither mineral salts nor vitamins release energy for use by the body. Energy is needed to perform chemical, physical and muscular work within the body and to produce the heat which provides the optimum conditions for life processes in the human. If the energy-producing foods (carbohydrates, fats and protein) are taken in excess of requirements, fat is stored and the individual puts on weight. If fat, carbohydrate and protein are taken in insufficient quantities, then the body stores of these substances are used, and weight is lost. The measure used to estimate an individual's requirement of these foods is the kilojoule (kJ). A kilojoule is one thousand joules. The unit of energy is the joule (J) and is the energy expended in moving one kilogram (kg) one metre (m) by a force of one newton (N). Until comparatively recently, the unit used to calculate energy intakes was the kilocalorie. This is usually referred to as the Calorie, written with a capital or upper case 'C' to distinguish it from the calorie, which is one-thousandth of a kilocalorie. Both Calorie values and kilojoule values are stated on food products. Energy requirements vary with the amount of muscular work carried out, the size of the individual, the age, and the efficiency with which the body stores and uses energy. A patient lying in bed will require fewer kilojoules than an active, working individual, but very restless patients, for instance after head injury, may use a gret deal of energy and require a relatively high energy intake. The average diet should contain about 15% of the energy in the form of protein, 50−60% in the form of carbohydrate, and 25−30% in the form of fat, of which only 10% should be in the form of saturated fatty acids.

Dietary fibre

Fibre is a term used to describe all the indigestible substances contained in food which pass unchanged through the digestive tract to emerge in the faeces. Typically, fibre is found in whole cereals, vegetables, fruit and nuts. Refined cereals have had a good deal of the fibre removed.

Water

All tissues in the body contain water in varying proportions. For instance, the teeth contain 5% water and bone 32% water. Other tissues contain a greater proportion of water than this, the greatest being the lungs which contain 84%. Urea and other waste products require water so that they may be excreted in solution. Water is required for the cooling of the body surface by sweat and for moistening inspired air. Digestive secretions contain a large volume of water, which is lost from the body if vomiting or diarrhoea occurs. Fluid is usually taken at meal times and it helps to dilute the food, giving a solution in which dietary enzymes can work easily. Food also needs to be moist to aid chewing, swallowing and taste. Most people also drink fluid of various kinds between meals. Water is absorbed into the body from the stomach and the intestines along with dissolved food molecules. It is also absorbed from the colon. Keeping fluid balance charts ensures that the patient gets sufficient fluid for his needs, and that fluid is neither retained nor excreted in excess.

HEALTHY EATING

There has recently been an upsurge of interest in 'healthy eating', but the idea of linking the type of food we eat with our state of health is one that goes back a long time. For example, in the sixteenth century the link between scurvy and a diet lacking fresh fruit and vegetables became apparent, and, by 1753, Lind had proved that scurvy could be cured by eating oranges and lemons.

Surprisingly, in Britain, the diet imposed by rationing during the Second World War (1939–1945) proved greatly beneficial in improving the health of the nation. This was shown by a sudden reduction in the perinatal death rate between 1940 and 1948 (DHSS, 1979). There was also a general increase in the height of the postwar generation over the pre-1930 generation by an average of 5 cm.

Over the past two or three decades there has arisen the view that the West suffers from 'diseases of affluence' due to eating over-refined foods, coupled with general overeating and/or an excessive intake of some types of nutrient. Among the diseases attributed to this are coronary heart disease, hypertension, diabetes mellitus, cholecystitis, diverticular disease and carcinoma of the colon.

The cause and effect relationship between deficiency diseases and diet is well established. Examples include rickets due to vitamin D deficiency, scurvy due to vitamin C deficiency, iron-deficiency anaemia, and kwashiorkor due to protein and total calorie deficiency. Similarly, the link between food contaminated with microorganisms and 'food poisoning' is clear-cut, as is the cause−effect relationship of illness or death and food contamination with chemically toxic substances, e.g. mercury, arsenic.

However, links between dietary intake and some of the diseases of affluence listed above is much less clear, making unequivocal dietary advice very difficult. There is no doubt that some advice given in the recent past and said to be based on firm scientific evidence is now suspect. An example is the advice during the 1950s to take very high protein diets in order to reduce obesity.

All we can do is to give advice in the light of the best scientific evidence available at the time. For example, dietary guidelines were issued by the DHSS (1979). These included a warning against obesity. Reduced intake of salt, protein, alcohol, fat and sugar was advocated, and the benefits of breast-feeding over bottle-feeding for infants were made clear. The National Advisory Committee on Nutrition Education (1983) issued advice which is still probably the most authoritative available, even though now somewhat outdated. They suggested that fat should form no higher proportion of the total energy intake than 30%, of which only 10% should be in the form of saturated fat. Less red meat should be eaten, and the total proportion of protein should be reduced. Sugar and salt intakes should be reduced, whilst fruit, vegetables and fibre intakes should be increased.

Apart from advice about salt reduction, most advice centres around issues of fibre and fat in food and the impact of obesity upon health. Heavy use of salt added to food is believed to be associated with the possible onset and/or maintenance of high blood pressure (hypertension). The relationship is a tenuous one since, physiologically, excessive salt absorbed into the body would be excreted provided kidney function were satisfactory.

Fibre

Fibre is known to be important as a part of the normal diet. It is found in unrefined cereals, vegetables, fruit and nuts. Fibre increases the bulk of food in proportion to its calorific value, such that, in general, the more fibre present, the lower the calorific value of any given weight of food. It follows that food high in fibre can satisfy an individual's appetite at a lower calorie value, thus helping to prevent obesity.

Fibre is not absorbed into the body from the intestinal tract. Its presence within the tract stimulates peristalsis and reduces the transit time of a meal from the moment of eating until the residue is excreted. This means that less water is absorbed from the tract, leaving faecal matter which is soft, bulky and more easily excreted, preventing constipation. This function of fibre can be of use in hospital to help to prevent the constipation which can occur amongst patients who are suddenly subjected to a more sedentary life-style. Bran may be added to breakfast cereals. However, a sudden increase in dietary fibre from a lower to a high level, may cause gastrointestinal discomfort and diarrhoea. Patients must therefore be assessed carefully and the amount of bran added to food should be calculated on an individual basis.

The rapid intestinal transit time associated with high

fibre diets is also believed to help in the prevention of diverticulitis and carcinoma of the colon, since these diseases may be associated with very slow transit times leaving food residues in the intestine or colon over long periods. There is also some evidence that diets high in fibre help to protect against coronary heart disease. The mechanism through which this protection could occur is by the promotion of increased cholesterol excretion.

Fat

Coronary heart disease is a condition in which atheromatous plaques formed on the lining of blood vessels reduce the internal diameter or calibre of the coronary arteries, putting the blood supply to the heart itself at risk. The problem may manifest itself in the form of angina, where the reduction in blood supply to the heart causes intense pain. A critically serious manifestation is that of myocardial infarction, where the blood supply within a coronary vessel is reduced to the level where it is cut off altogether. The section of heart muscle supplied by this vessel then dies. Myocardial infarction is a major cause of premature death in Western societies in general, and in the UK in particular. Here the rate is higher than in most other Western countries. The condition is one that is particularly prevalent from middle-age onward. In middle-age, men are at greater risk than women, but amongst the elderly the risk is more evenly distributed between the sexes.

The best evidence currently available links a sedentary life-style and a diet high in cholesterol and saturated fatty acids with a predisposition to the development of atheroma. Smoking also plays an important role in the development of myocardial infarction. Consequently, those at risk are advised to reduce their intake of foods containing saturated fatty acids and cholesterol. These foods include red meat, eggs and dairy products made from whole milk or cream. Those with sedentary occupations are also advised to include exercise in their daily or weekly routines. Since it is difficult to pinpoint precisely those at risk of developing atheroma, the advice is that everyone should reduce the intake of foods containing saturated fat from an early age.

It should be noted that coronary heart disease is not the only problem that may arise from atheroma. Strokes due either to thrombosis within intracranial arteries or to intracerebral haemorrhage may occur as a result of atheroma. These tend to occur in a more elderly section of the population than coronary heart disease. Stroke is a condition of high prevalence in this country, and if the individual survives the stroke, they are frequently severely disabled.

A diet which is high in fat can also contribute to obesity. Obesity predisposes to hypertension, which in itself increases the risk of a stroke.

Other factors contributing to a healthy diet

From what has been said above, an individual who wishes to reduce their fat intake may well cut down on whole milk products. However, milk and food processed from milk are good sources of calcium. Calcium is required by the body to develop and maintain the structure of bone and teeth. This is in addition to its role in blood clotting and its importance in the promotion of normal nerve impulses and muscular contraction (including heart muscle). Clearly the latter function is essential to life. If total calcium levels within the body are low, homeostatic mechanisms take calcium from the bone to maintain the blood, nerve and muscle levels. Under such circumstances bone becomes fragile.

Dietary calcium intake is important in babies and children when bone is developing and growing, in pregnant women, in people with fractures and in the elderly. An increasing cause of admission to hospital among the elderly in the UK is fractured neck of femur. This is associated with low trauma. In some cases it is believed to occur spontaneously and is due to a condition called osteoporosis. Osteoporosis is a condition where the density of bone is reduced due to loss of calcium. It occurs in the elderly and in women more than men. It is associated with a drop in hormonal levels in the postmenopausal woman. The condition is also linked with absence of exercise. Osteoporosis causes vertebral fractures and Colles' fractures, but these occur in a 'younger' elderly population than fractured neck of femur and are less serious.

Whilst the administration of calcium cannot reverse the condition, it can be seen that it is important to maintain a good intake amongst those at risk. Due to the importance of calcium, people are advised not to cut out milk and its products but to change to the use of skimmed milk, low fat yoghurts and cheeses.

Amongst other essential minerals, the diet may be deficient in iron; this will cause iron-deficiency anaemia. A normal diet will contain enough iron for the average requirement. However, women who have heavy menstrual periods may need an increase in dietary iron, which can be found in red meat, liver and green vegetables.

Food poisoning from microorganisms is still a problem in the UK. Infants and the elderly are at risk from severe illness or even death. It is important that strict hygiene is maintained in food preparation and handling. People are also advised not to reheat food which has already been cooked, and not to allow any contact between uncooked and cooked food. Clearly all food must be cooked for a sufficient time at the correct temperature to kill micro-organisms.

Increasingly today, people are concerned about food additives in manufactured and convenience foods. This is partly because such additives are labelled with a number which has no meaning for most people and so they are confronted with a 'mystery' ingredient. Also there are worries that some food additives may be carcinogenic if taken over a long period of time. However, it should be stated that scientific testing is carried out on food additives and only 'safe' additives are allowed for use.

Perhaps more worrying to the general population is the question of pesticides and herbicides used in the production of food, since these often remain active over long periods of time and get incorporated within the structure of the vegetable, fruit or animal concerned. It may then be differentially distributed within a structure, and/or concentrated during storage and still be present in food.

Advice from nurses to those who are worried should be up to date, taking account of all the evidence available. Greater precautions to ensure the safety of food need to be taken in relation to those who are particularly vulnerable. These are the very young, pregnant women, the elderly and those who already have a physiological problem. The question of healthy eating is complex. However, to sum up, a good balanced diet is one which contains all the essential nutrients, has high levels of fibre, is low in saturated fatty acids and cholesterol, low in sugar and has little added salt, but contains plenty of fresh fruit, vegetables and cereal products.

Fried foods are best avoided or eaten in very low

quantities, using vegetable oil as the cooking agent. In total, the calorie intake should balance the physical activity level to prevent obesity. In maintaining weight at the optimum level it is better to take exercise than to take a very low calorific diet and no exercise.

NUTRITIONAL NEEDS OF HOSPITAL PATIENTS

It is a common belief that Western society suffers from 'diseases of affluence' (see above). It is surprising, therefore, that surveys have identified protein calorie malnutrition (PCM) in a number of hospital patients, both amongst medical patients and patients admitted for surgery (Hill et al, 1977; Coates, 1982). Malnutrition is defined as a pathological state resulting from a relative or absolute deficiency or excess of one or more essential nutrients. Protein calorie malnutrition describes a state in which there is a depletion of the body's protein, most of which, it will be recalled, is incorporated into cell structure, plasma protein, etc. When food intake is insufficient to supply energy needs, stores of energy in the form of fat and glycogen are depleted, then protein is split down and its constituent amino acids are converted into glucose or lipid molecules and used.

It is not difficult to understand that patients might be malnourished on admission to hospital. Indeed, they may have been admitted precisely because of symptoms of loss of appetite, vomiting, diarrhoea, or signs of weight loss. What is less easy to understand is that the condition may deteriorate further in hospital.

It is well documented that surgical patients are frequently starved preoperatively for much longer periods than is necessary (Smith, 1974; Royal College of Physicians, 1989). Meals may be missed due to investigations or treatments; facilities are now rarely available for providing light meals from ward kitchens to substitute for missed meals.

Meals may be distributed to patients and plates cleared away by domestic staff with no involvement at all by nurses. Nurses may therefore be completely unaware of patients who have left food portions uneaten. Patients who need to be helped with eating may also lose out.

A frequent assumption is that patients in hospital are sedentary and therefore do not have high calorie requirements. However, injury, infection and some disease processes increase the metabolic rate and therefore energy requirements. The normal hospital diet may fail to fulfil these increased energy requirements.

Any hospital catering department must provide for a large number of people. Athough a choice of menu is provided, patients must frequently make this choice some hours in advance. Patients with a poor appetite may not then feel tempted by the food they fancied some hours previously.

Clearly, the first step in helping both to prevent and to reverse malnutrition is the recognition of the problem. Good nutritional assessment is essential.

Nutritional assessment

There are many methods of nutritional assessment but no one method is adequate on its own. Some techniques are complex and beyond the scope of this book.

Methods can be classified into four broad groups (Moghissi and Boore, 1983).

1. Obtaining information directly from the patient by interview or questionnaire.
2. Physical examination including anthropometry.
3. Biochemical tests.

4. Tests of immune function.

Another method which should be mentioned is direct observation of a patient's food intake, since nurses are in a good position to carry this out.

Interview with the patient

A nutritional history is frequently collected by health professionals other than nurses (e.g. doctors, dieticians). The nurse will normally collect a nutritional history as part of the nursing history on admission or shortly afterwards. This includes information relevant to the patient's normal diet and current nutritional state. At least some of the following details will be obtained during interview.

1. Whether or not the patient's appetite has changed recently. If it has, one enquires in what way it has changed and whether he can think of a reason for the change.
2. In the patient's opinion, is his appetite large, small, or average in comparison with mates at work, friends, relatives, etc.
3. Whether or not the patient has lost or gained weight recently.
4. Does the patient ever get pain related to food and, if so, what is the nature and timing of the pain.
5. Normally, does the patient have a small number of large meals or a greater number of small meals in the day.
6. Any foods known to cause upset should be recorded.
7. Tactful enquiry may be made as to whether the diet normally contains whole foods, convenience foods, and how varied it is.
8. Note is taken of whether the patient is on any special diet and whether this is from preference or for religious or medical reasons.

9. The approximate normal fluid intake should be recorded.
10. Any difficulty in swallowing or chewing should be noted.
11. Information about the bowel action is also relevant.

Note. It is sometimes suggested that a patient should be asked about the times at which meals are normally taken. I suggest that this should be omitted unless it is of particular relevance, since meal times in hospital are fixed. To ask questions about meal times may lead to a false expectation that the nurse can adapt the times to special needs.

A good deal of nutritional information can be gained by the skilled nurse through unobtrusive observation during interview. Note should be taken of the condition of the patient's hair, skin and eyes. The colour of the skin and mucous membranes should be noted, together with any signs of soreness of the lips or corners of the mouth. Rapid turnover of the cells of skin and mucous membrane may reveal signs of malnutrition. Any obesity or undernourishment should be noted. If there appears any cause for concern, then closer examination of the tongue, skinfold thickness, etc., can follow.

Recording body weight

Body weight is one of the most convenient of the anthropometric measures. It is a useful indicator of nutritional status and it is recommended that all patients should have their body weight recorded on admission. This is useful not only in relation to nutritional status but also as an indicator for dosage of drugs and anaesthetics. Clearly the measure is of little benefit unless it is accurate and the scales which are used should therefore be tested for their accuracy at frequent intervals and should be well maintained. The condition under which the weight was measured should be recorded together with the weight; for example, the exact clothing worn, the interval since the last meal, the time of day and date. The patient should have been asked to empty the bladder before the weight was recorded. The presence of any oedema should be noted.

A single recording of weight is not necessarily helpful in nutritional assessment by itself; it requires interpretation in the light of (1) standard weight/height tables and (2) the patient's usual weight.

The nursing care plan

The nursing care plan will be written on the basis of the nursing history and assessment followed by the identification of any existing or potential nutritional problems. The means to overcome or prevent problems will be identified as part of the plan. Objectives of care may include teaching the patient nutritional principles as a means of maintaining health. Instructions for nursing care may include observing the amount of food the patient eats, encouraging him to eat, or to stick to a reducing diet. Any deviation from the normal diet provided by the hospital kitchen, which is part of the patient's care, must be included on the care plan.

FEEDING PATIENTS IN HOSPITAL

Patients' diets in hospital, other than those ordered individually from the special diet kitchen, are often classed as 'full', 'light' and 'fluid'. A patient taking full diet usually has three main meals (breakfast, midday dinner and supper) and the food served will be similar to that which he is accustomed to eat at home. Apart from therapeutic diets, some special diets may be needed for patients whose racial or religious customs may prohibit the eating of certain foods; for example, the kosher diet of the Jewish people, and strictly vegetarian diets. Light diet commonly includes eggs, fish and chicken with additional milk drinks between main meals. Fluid diets, of which the basis is usually milk and sweetened fruit drinks, are generally served at 2-hourly intervals.

Some of the difficulties encountered in catering for large numbers are the distances which the cooked food has to travel between the central kitchen and the wards, and the need to cook some food a considerable time before it will be eaten. The proper planning of kitchens and the provision of adequate equipment help to solve this latter problem. Trolleys with separate compartments for hot and cold foods are in general use for the transport of food to the wards. In some hospitals a tray system whereby individual meals are served directly on to the patients' trays in the kitchen and then conveyed immediately to the ward has been introduced. Special plates are used to keep hot food at the correct temperature.

Most hospitals have a catering manager who considers all aspects of providing food for patients and staff, buying supplies, approving dietary scales and arrangements for cooking and serving meals. Special therapeutic diets, for example diabetic, reducing or low energy, high protein, calcium balance diets, are planned and supervised by a qualified dietitian.

Serving meals

The practice as regards serving meals may vary in different hospitals but the nurse needs to be aware of the patient's food preferences and to observe the amount of food a patient actually eats. Eating is a pleasure for the great majority of people, and meals should be so presented that they are occasions to which the patients look forward. Thus they should be served attractively and at the right temperature. Individual tastes should be considered so that, for example, gravy is not automatically put on to every plate regardless of whether a patient likes it or not. If the patient really cannot tolerate the meal sent from the kitchen, effort should be made to provide an alternative, even if this entails cooking a simple meal such as scrambled egg in the ward kitchen. The nurse should position her patients so that they can eat their meals in comfort. Dirty china should be cleared away immediately, especially if food scraps are left on the plate. Cold congealed, half-eaten food can be most unpleasant for sensitive but well individuals, let alone ill ones.

Feeding patients

Skill, patience and gentleness are needed to feed another individual successfully with food or fluid. The speed with which a patient eats needs to be observed, so that the nurse matches this with the rate at which the food is presented. The nurse needs to be able to place the spoon or fork accurately into the patient's mouth; if it is placed too far back it may produce gagging. If the movements of patient and nurse are not coordinated, the spoon or fork may hit against the patient's tongue or teeth and cause discomfort. Some people like to eat one kind of food at a time, whilst others like several different kinds of food mixed together. Patients may find it difficult to swallow unless they have frequent sips of water, whilst others do not like cold fluid while they are eating hot food. A sip of water can act as a boundary between two different types of food, and to go straight from a savoury food such as fish to a sweet food, or from a greasy food to a non-greasy food, without the opportunity to rinse the mouth with water, can be extremely distasteful. Such preferences must be taken into account. The nurse should sit down when feeding a patient so that this is made a pleasant social occasion.

If a patient with a neurological lesion is being fed, then careful observation must be made to detect any difficulty in swallowing. The swallowing reflex can be initiated by gentle pressure on the tongue with the spoon. Care must be taken to feed the patient from the side of the face on which there is no weakness or sensory loss, and to ensure that food does not accumulate in the cheek on the affected side.

When blind patients are being fed, it is important that they are told exactly what food is being given them, to avoid the shock of expecting one taste and getting a different type of food. If possible, even with blind patients, it is better if the patient can actually place the food in the mouth for himself, even though the nurse has placed the food on to the spoon or fork.

An angled straw, used with a cup or drinking glass, may be used to give drinks to helpless patients. If a spouted feeding cup is used, then the patient should be told he can put his tongue over the end of the spout to control the flow; otherwise he may be afraid of choking. The best way to support the head while the patient is drinking is to put an arm under the pillow, raising the pillow and the head together.

When children are admitted into hospital, it is a good idea to ask about their special likes and dislikes with respect to food, and also about the way in which they normally eat their food. If their normal diet is totally unsuitable, they may be coaxed into eating more suitable food, but it must be remembered that the child will be returning to the environment from which he came.

Tube feeding

If a patient is unable to swallow for any reason, he may be fed artificially using a tube passed down the oesophagus into the stomach. Conditions in which tube feeding may be necessary are:

1. Coma.
2. Paralysis of the soft palate or pharyngeal muscle.
3. After operation on the mouth, pharynx or larynx.
4. For premature or weak infants who are unable to suck.

Principles

1. Great care must be taken before any fluid is given to ensure that the tube is correctly placed in the stomach, and is neither in the lungs, nor coiled in the mouth or pharynx. Two people should check the position of the tube, and in some hospitals it is required that one of these should be a qualified nurse or doctor.
2. Air should not be allowed to enter the stomach whilst the feed is being given; therefore the apparatus should not be allowed to become empty until the entire feed has been administered.
3. To avoid discomfort caused by the sudden stimulation of stomach nerve endings by cold fluid, the feed should be warmed to body temperature, 37°C (98.6°F), and tested with a lotion thermometer before it is given.
4. Sudden distension of the stomach can also stimulate nerve endings and cause discomfort. This can be avoided by giving the feed slowly, either by the use of small apparatus or by pinching the tube slightly as the food is given, to reduce its calibre.
5. It is not necessary to remove the tube after every feed

if it has been passed nasally, but it will require periodic removal for cleaning and to avoid a tissue reaction. A rubber tube should be changed every 24 hours, a polythene one every 7 days.

6. Lack of skill in passing a tube into the stomach can cause damage to the mucous membrane of the nose, nasopharynx or oesophagus. If any difficulty is encountered, the attempt to pass the tube should be abandoned. A later attempt, by a different individual, or using different apparatus, may be more successful.

Requirements

- Mouthwash, *or* tray for cleaning the mouth, if the tube is to be passed orally
- Orange sticks and wool swabs; a gallipot containing sodium bicarbonate, for cleaning the nostrils if the tube is to be passed nasally
- Small glass or polythene funnel
- Oesophageal tube (Figure 7.1), size 6 to 18 (English gauge) or 14 to 22 (French gauge). (The larger sizes are used for the oral route, the smaller for the nasal route.)
- Bowl for the apparatus
- Measure containing water, to clear the tube
- Measure containing the feed
- Lotion thermometer
- Protective cape and a towel
- 30 ml of water to clear the tube before and after the feed
- Liquid paraffin *or* water to act as a lubricant
- 50-ml syringe and an adaptor
- Measure and litmus paper, for gastric juice
- Disposable plastic gloves
- *For an unconscious patient*, a tray containing a tongue

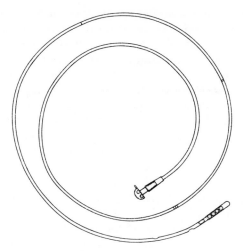

Figure 7.1 Oesophageal tube.

spatula, tongue forceps and a gag should be provided, so that the mouth may be opened to observe the position of the tube

Passing the tube

First of all, the procedure must be explained to the patient in language he will understand. He should be told:

1. The reason for the procedure.
2. Approximately how long it will take.
3. What it will feel like.
4. What he has to do to help.

The nasal route. Position the patient, sitting him up well with the head slightly flexed if possible. Put on the plastic gloves. Clean the nostrils and observe if the nasal septum is deviated from the midline. Note, as a guide the approximate distance of 50—60 cm from the stomach end of the tube before the tube is inserted. Pass the tube gently along the floor of the larger nostril. In older patients the shape of the nose alters and the tube should be directed in a rather more downward path than is the case for a younger person. Ask the patient to swallow as the tube is passed down the oesophagus. Proceed slowly, and do not persist if there is any resistance to the passage of the tube. A conscious patient will cough if the tube enters the larynx, and the tube must be withdrawn. A deeply unconscious patient will have no cough reflex but he may become cyanosed if the tube enters the respiratory system. The tube should be in the stomach when it has passed for 50—62 cm, depending upon the height of the adult.

The oral route. Any dentures should be removed. The procedure is the same as for the nasal route, except that the tube is passed over the tongue, not through a nostril. A mouth gag may be needed to hold open the mouth of an unconscious patient.

Checking that the tube is in the stomach

There are two ways of checking that the tube is in the stomach.

1. A syringe is attached to the end of the tube and a specimen of fluid obtained by suction. This is tested by litmus paper for acidity, since gastric juice has a low pH (it contains hydrochloric acid). If there is any difficulty in obtaining a specimen of gastric juice it may be helpful to place the patient in the left lateral position with one pillow under the head, and the foot of the bed on blocks. This helps the gastric fluid to gravitate to the fundus of the stomach, where it has been shown that the end of the tube tends to lie.

2. The other method of ensuring that the tube is in the correct place is by placing a stethoscope over the stomach and listening through the ear pieces whilst 5 ml air is injected through the stomach tube, using a Dakin's or 50-ml syringe. If the end of the tube is in the stomach, the air will be heard, by means of the stethoscope, as it enters.

Note. Another method for checking the position of the tube is sometimes proposed. This consists of connecting a funnel and tubing on to the tube, inverting the funnel into a bowl of water, and observing for the presence or absence of bubbles from the apparatus. The presence of bubbles signifies that the tube is in the respiratory tract. In my opinion, this is a very bad method to use for two reasons.

1. If the tube is in the respiratory tract, the patient will be breathing in as well as out, and on inspiration the fluid will be sucked up into the apparatus. If a small funnel and short tubing are used, there is a real danger that this fluid may get into the patient's respiratory tract.
2. A demonstration that the tube is *not* in the respiratory tract does not show that it *is* in the stomach. Thus the methods discussed above are safer as regards ensuring that the tube is in the stomach.

Preparation of the feed

Ideally the dietary requirements for each patient who is being tube fed should be drawn up by the dietitian. The prescribed requirements can then be translated into pre-pared liquids containing the correct amount of fluid and nutrients to maintain the patient's body weight, hydration and nutritional status. Such liquid diets, sent from the diet kitchen and carefully labelled, should be divided into suitable amounts and frequency in the 24 hours to ensure that each patient obtains his full prescription. The nurse then only needs to warm the fluid to the correct temperature, 37°C (98.6°F), and to administer the correct amount, carefully measured, and on time.

However, it is by no means always the case that such facilities are available within a hospital. In the absence of such facilities, the responsibility for ensuring that each patient's body weight, nutritional status and fluid balance are maintained seems to devolve upon the ward sister or charge nurse (Jones, 1975), who may (and should) seek advice from the dietitian in planning the dietary needs of each patient. The sister or charge nurse will also carry out an assessment of the patient's condition and activity level. The diet should then be clearly written down to form part of the care plan or Kardex record. Diet sheets should be posted in the ward kitchen. If the feed is to be prepared in the ward, then the sheet should state:

1. The product to be used, e.g. Complan.
2. The amount of the product in grams.
3. The type of fluid to be used, e.g. milk, milk and water, or water.
4. The amount of additional fluid needed by the patient to maintain hydration.

Tables of recommended allowances prepared by the DHSS (1979) should be available in the ward kitchen, as should the composition of any frequently used feed, e.g. Complan.

The nurse in charge should give clear and unambiguous instructions about preparation of the feed when asking someone to do this. If the instructions are not clear, the nurse who is to carry out the procedure should seek clarification.

The following *equipment* is required.

1. Graduated measures and containers for liquids are needed, together with an accurate balance for weighing small amounts of powder.
2. Proprietary feeds should be stored in the manufacturer's containers with the information about content and instructions for preparation on the outside. Instructions for mixing and diluting such feeds must be carefully followed.

The feed should be *prepared* with regard to the following points.

1. All ingredients should be accurately measured according to the instructions on the diet sheet.
2. Instructions for diluting mixtures from the diet kitchen or main kitchen should be followed carefully.
3. Manufacturers' instructions for preparation of feeds should be followed. A small amount of fluid should be carefully added to the Complan powder and the two should be mixed in a mixer. The resulting solution can then be further diluted with the remainder of the prescribed fluid. If no mixer is available, a small amount of fluid should be added to the powder in a cup and the two whisked with a fork. When all the powder has dissolved and no lumps remain, the mixture can be diluted with the remainder of the liquid. Using either of these methods there should be no lumps. If any appear they should be broken down and added to the feed. They must never be discarded without being replaced, otherwise the patient is being starved of a portion of his diet.
4. Equipment for use should be assembled and liquids put on to heat before dry products are weighed.
5. The temperature of the feed (37°C, 98.6°F) should be

estimated with a lotion thermometer kept for this purpose in the kitchen.

Note: This section on preparation of tube feeds is based on Jones (1975). Readers are advised to refer to his book *Food for Thought* for more information on this topic.

Method of administration of the feed

Having checked the position of the tube, the temperature of the fluid is checked and a funnel is attached to the end of the tube. Some tubing may be interposed between the oesophageal tube and the funnel, if necessary. Half of the water is inserted into the funnel and allowed to enter the stomach before the feed, ensuring easier flow of the thicker liquid. The feed is run in slowly; the tube may be pinched if necessary. The funnel should not be allowed to empty or air will enter the stomach. At the end of the feed, the remaining water is used to clear the tube and the tube is either spigotted and attached to the patient's forehead or it is pinched, and gently withdrawn. If the tube is not pinched as it is withdrawn, any fluid remaining in it will empty, and may drop into the larynx causing choking or chest infection, depending upon whether the cough reflex is present or not.

Following the administration of the feed, the details should be entered on to the fluid chart, e.g. Complan 50 g + water 180 ml.

Aspiration of the stomach

Stomach aspiration is carried out by the nursing staff; it is not a sterile procedure, although sterile equipment may be used. The stomach may be aspirated hourly to rest the alimentary tract in paralytic ileus, or after an operation on the alimentary tract.

Once the tube is in place it may remain in position for 24 hours at a time, provided it has been passed nasally.

Requirements

- 20-ml syringe and an adaptor
- Measure for the aspirated fluid
- Sterile spigot
- Adhesive tape
- Fluid chart
- Polythene sheet and paper towel
- Plastic disposable gloves

Method

Protect the patient's chest. Put on the plastic gloves. Remove the tube from the patient's cheek. This should have been fastened to the cheek by adhesive tape in such a way that the tube can be slipped away without the tape having to be removed from the skin every time.

Special clips for attaching the tube to the forehead are available commercially and are frequently used. Remove the spigot and attach the syringe to the end of the tube, using the adaptor. Apply suction to the tube by drawing on the piston of the syringe. Pinch the tubing and disconnect the syringe when it is full. Empty into the measure, re-attach and repeat until no more fluid is obtained. Insert the fresh spigot, re-attach the tube to the cheek and leave the patient comfortable. Record the amount and nature of the aspirant.

8   Ensuring patient comfort

One of the daily living activities a nurse undertakes for a patient is to make the bed, or to ensure that it is made by an assistant.

BEDMAKING

Skilled bedmaking, placing pillows comfortably and correct positioning, contributes a good deal to the comfort of an ill person who will spend the greater part of the time in bed.

Principles of bedmaking

1. Bedmaking should be carried out as often as is necessary to keep the patient comfortable and to make sure that the sheets are smooth and clean, but at the same time an ill patient should not be disturbed merely to ensure that the bed looks tidy.
2. The quality of the mattress is to some extent beyond the nurse's control, but she should at least make sure that mattresses are replaced when they become worn, and that the patient gets the most suitable type of mattress.
3. Cross-infection is a danger if bedmaking is carried out unskilfully. Movement of the bedclothes dislodges microorganisms from the bed into the air and also disturbs the air above the bed, increasing the area over which microorganisms may be airborne. Excess shaking and flapping of the bedclothes should be

avoided, and smooth movements causing little disturb-ance of the air should be used.

4. The bedclothes should be stripped on to a chair which is used exclusively for the patient, or on to a bed stripper attached as an integral part of the patient's bed. A bed stripper, carried from bed to bed, is a potential danger from the cross-infection point of view. Care should be taken to prevent the bedclothes from dragging on to the floor, picking up microorganisms; passers-by should be careful not to brush the bedclothes with their personal clothing.

5. Bedclothes should never be stripped completely from over the patient, leaving him uncovered. A sheet should be left in place if the ward temperature is warm, or a blanket if it is cold. Patient comfort should be the prime concern whilst the bed is being made; if a patient is being turned, or moved, it must be done very gently and a pillow left under the head for comfort.

6. If the patient is hot and sticky, ensure that the sheets are replaced so that a cool, fresh area is in contact with the patient.

7. All the equipment which may be required should be available at the bedside, before stripping the bed, and two people should work together so that the bed is made as efficiently and quickly as possible and the patient moved without causing pain or excessive exertion.

8. Removal of debris from the sheets and tautening creases from the sheets help to prevent pressure sores.

9. The mattress should be pulled well up to the bedhead.

To make an occupied bed

1. Explain to the patient that the bed is to be made.
2. Place the chair at the foot of the bed if there is not a

bed-stripping area incorporated into the bedstead. Loosen the bedclothes on either side and from the foot of the mattress.

3. Starting at the top of the bed, move towards the foot of the bed, taking the counterpane from the top and folding it neatly into three or four as you go, and finally lay it on the chair or stripper. If it is likely to drag on the floor, fold the sides up neatly over the chair to prevent this.

4. Repeat with the other top bedclothes except for a sheet or blanket, which is used to cover the patient, maintaining warmth and dignity.

5. Remove all but one pillow and place on to a chair near the head of the bed, whilst one nurse supports the patient.

6. Roll the patient to one side, placing one pillow under the head. The nurse towards whom the patient faces should stand close to the bed, so the patient does not feel afraid of falling out.

7. Roll the draw sheet and polythene sheeting to the centre of the bed (Figure 8.1).

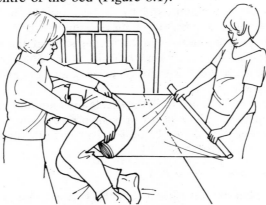

Figure 8.1 A disposable waterproof sheet in use.

8. If the bottom sheet needs changing, roll this also to the centre of the bed and tuck in the new sheet on one side and halfway along the head and foot of the mattress. Use the folds laundered into the sheet to ensure that it is centred properly. Make sure that a good amount is tucked in at the bottom. Roll up the other half of the sheet lengthways in the middle of the bed. Bring back the polythene over the top of the roll and also the draw sheet unless a clean one is inserted. If the bottom sheet is not being changed, it should be untucked, brushed clean with the hand and tucked in again, so that no creases remain, pulling it up well, before smoothing and tucking in the polythene and draw sheet.

9. Roll the patient gently on to the opposite side, taking the precaution mentioned above. Warn about any sheets rolled in the middle of the bed, since these will give the feeling of a big 'hump'.

10. Remove all dirty sheets into a container at the bedside. Smooth the sheets, brush all debris away, and tuck them in as smoothly and tightly as possible; thus the making of the bottom of the bed is completed.

11. Turn the patient back to the centre of the bed and give support whilst the pillows are 'plumped' and rearranged. Lift him into a comfortable position.

12. As soon as the top sheet has been placed over the patient, the covering blanket may be removed. Replace the top bedclothes.

13. Ensure that the bedclothes are loose over the patient's feet. A bed cradle may be used to support their weight but, in the absence of this, the bedclothes should be pleated over the feet, or the patient can be asked to cross one foot over the other whilst the bed is being made, ensuring plenty of room for the feet.

14. Replace the patient's locker in a convenient position.

An alternative method

If the condition of the patient allows, it may be easier to lift the patient to the foot of the bed where he can be supported by one nurse. The bottom sheets at the head of the bed are straightened or changed. The patient is then lifted back on to the newly made part of the bed whilst the lower ends of the bottom sheets are attended to.

To make a cot

A cot can be made easily by one nurse, since usually the child can be taken out of the cot and held on a nurse's knee. The procedure for making a cot is the same as that for making a bed, except that the counterpane is tucked in all round to allow the cot sides to be put up. A toddler may spend the greater part of the day on top of the bedclothes rather than in the bed, so should be warmly clothed. For safety, the cot sides must be fastened in position before the child is left.

To make the top bedclothes into a 'pack'

This is done whenever the patient is to be moved directly from a stretcher to the bed. Circumstances in which this might happen are:

1. On emergency admission.
2. On return to the ward from the operating theatre.
3. Following X-ray or any other examination in a separate department.

Method

Place the bottom sheet and draw sheet in position in the usual way. The top bedclothes are made up as usual at the head end of the bed but are left loose at the foot, allowing the usual amount for tuck in. When all the bedclothes have been replaced, the counterpane is folded back at the foot, the blankets are folded over it and finally the sheet. This allows for quick and easy tucking in when the patient is back in bed. The bedclothes are then folded so that they can be easily removed to allow the patient to be lifted on to the bed. An electric blanket may be placed in the bed to keep it warm.

Clean bed-linen should be used when making up the bed for a patient in the operating theatre; the bed frame itself and the mattress should have been cleaned with antiseptic and dried.

In the case of an emergency admission, if the patient is admitted fully clothed, or has been involved in a road traffic accident, the sheets may be protected by blankets, but it is cheaper and easier to launder sheets than blankets so this is not a very logical procedure.

Modifications of basic bedmaking in special conditions

After tonsillectomy

After this operation the patient will be nursed in a semi-prone position, with no pillow under the head (Figure 8.2). A pillow is placed under the mattress at the back of the patient to help maintain this position, and the top of the bed is protected by a disposable polythene sheet and draw sheet. A bed elevator should be available.

A divided bed

If traction is applied to a lower limb, a divided bed is used. A fracture board should be in position. The top bedclothes are made up in two sections by folding the blankets to the required size within a sheet; one section is

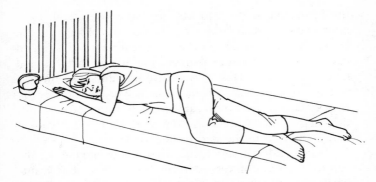

Figure 8.2 Position following tonsillectomy. Blood and secretions can drain easily from the mouth, preventing their inhalation.

to cover the patient's body, the other covers the good leg and tucks in at the foot of the bed. The limb to which traction has been applied emerges from between the two sections and should be covered by a small blanket.

Following amputation of the lower limb

A fracture board is required when a lower limb has been amputated and a divided bed (as described for traction applied to a lower limb) may be used, but more usually the bed is made up in the normal way over a bed cradle.

To allow drying of plaster of Paris

A good circulation of air around the wet plaster of Paris aids drying. For an upper limb, no modification of the bed is required. The limb should be supported on a firm, plastic-covered pillow on top of the bedclothes. In the case of a lower limb, a large bed cradle is used and the bedclothes are turned back over it so that the bed end is open to the air.

Sitting position

See Figure 8.3.

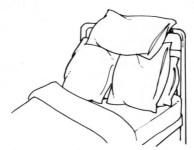

Figure 8.3 Bed prepared to support a patient in the sitting position. A patient with a drainage tube in the thoracic cavity connected with an underwater seal bottle will need a central gap between the almost vertically placed pillows. This is more comfortable and prevents kinking and obstruction of the tube.

POSITIONS USED IN NURSING

The nursing care plan may specify that the patient is to be nursed in a particular position. If such a position is not specified, the position chosen will be one of maximum comfort for the patient.

Upright position

The upright position is comfortable for the patient who is in bed during the daytime, when no other position is indicated (Figure 8.4). It is also a useful position to aid breathing and prevent chest complications.

Orthopnoeic position

The orthopnoeic position may be used in heart failure when the patient has great difficulty in breathing, unless

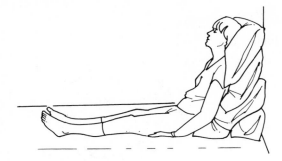

Figure 8.4 Upright position.

sitting well upright (Figure 8.5). He should be helped to
stay in position by means of a foot support (Figure 8.6).
This will help to prevent bed sores caused by a shearing
force as the patient slips down the bed. An arm rest can
be provided, as illustrated in Figure 8.5, by means of a
pillow placed on a bed table, enabling the patient to lean
forward.

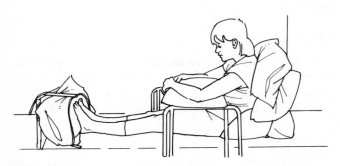

Figure 8.5 Orthopnoeic position.

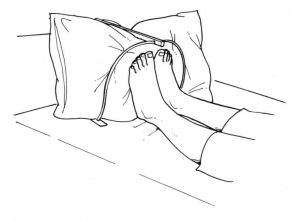

Figure 8.6 A foot support in use.

Recumbent position

In a recumbent position the patient lies flat with two pillows, at the most (Figure 8.7). This position is rarely used nowadays but may be employed if a patient has a low blood pressure.

Lateral position

The lateral position (Figure 8.8) is more commonly used if a patient must be flat for any reason. There is less danger of chest infection or pressure sores if the patient

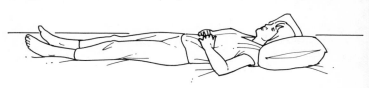

Figure 8.7 Recumbent position.

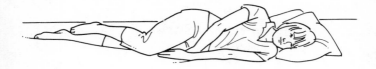

Figure 8.8 Lateral position.

can have his position changed from side to side. Besides this, the patient can see more of the ward activities in this position than in the recumbent position. Note that the lower arm rests in front of the patient and the upper leg rests on a pillow behind the lower leg.

Semi-prone position

A semi-prone position is one in which an unconscious patient is often nursed (Figure 8.9). It may also be used for gynaecological examination. In the case of an unconscious patient in whom the corneal reflex is absent, care should be taken to protect the eye from the pillow. Often there is no pillow used under the head of an unconscious patient for this reason. Note here that the lower arm is resting on the bed *behind* the patient, thus tilting the thorax and head so that fluid should drain from the mouth. The upper leg may be supported on a pillow in front of the lower leg.

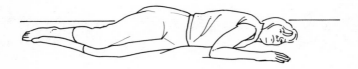

Figure 8.9 Semi-prone position.

Prone position

To relieve pressure if the sacral area and hips show signs of pressure, the prone position may be used (Figure 8.10). Note the supporting pillows beneath the upper abdomen, preventing lordosis of the spine. The pillows support the patient so that no part of the body rests on the mattress. It is especially important to use a sufficient number of pillows under the shins to prevent foot drop.

Dorsal position

The dorsal position is used for gynaecological examinations (Figure 8.11).

LIFTING THE PATIENT

Patients who are seriously ill or disabled will need to be moved within the bed or from chair to bed by the nursing staff. Lifting patients is a very skilled task and should be practised with friends as 'patients' before trying to lift real patients. There are two main considerations: one is the comfort of the patient, and the other is to make sure that the lift is properly executed so the nurse is caused no strain or damage in the process. An important rule to remember is that the thigh muscles, not the back muscles,

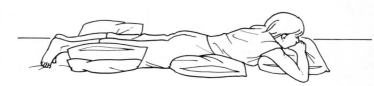

Figure 8.10   Prone position.

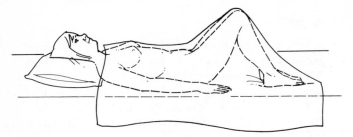

Figure 8.11 Dorsal position (gynaecological).

should be used to help lifting. The diagrams that follow (Figures 8.12–8.19) are an aid to learning how to lift but are no substitute for supervised practice.

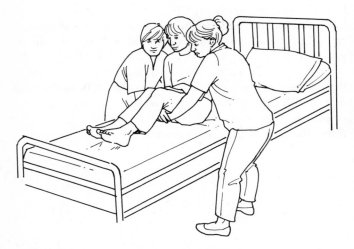

Figure 8.12 Orthodox lift. Lifting the patient up the bed. I. Note the position of the lifters' hands under the patient's thighs.

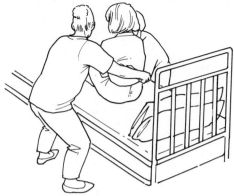

Figure 8.13 Orthodox lift. Lifting the patient up the bed. II. Note the position of the lifters' feet and legs and the posture of the head and back. Also note the position of the lifters' hands in relation to the patient's sacrum. The patient is moved by the lifters straightening their legs a little and transferring their weight in the direction of the movement.

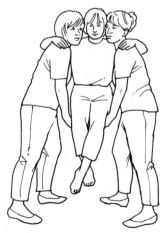

Figure 8.14 Orthodox lift. Lifting the patient from bed to chair. Note particularly the bent knees of the lifters, and the positions of their feet. The lifters' hands support the small of the patient's back.

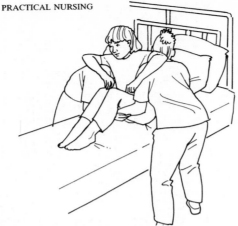

Figure 8.15 Shoulder lift. Lifting the patient up the bed. I. Starting position. Note the general position of the lifters in relation to the patient. It is essential that the lifters stand level with the patient's hips. One lifter grasps the other's forearm under the patient's thighs, and each presses her shoulder into the patient's axilla. The patient should be asked to rest the arms lightly on the lifters' backs.

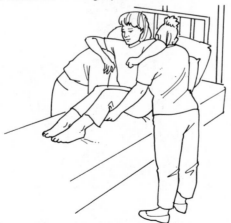

Figure 8.16 Shoulder lift. Lifting the patient up the bed. II. The lift. Having pressed her shoulder into the patient's axilla, each lifter smoothly extends her hips and knees and transfers her weight on to the forward leg. Throughout the movement the lifters stand as close to the bed as possible. Note that the shoulder lift cannot be used if the patient has injuries to the upper part of the trunk, shoulder or arms.

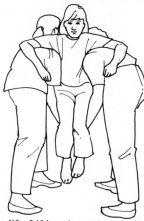

Figure 8.17 Shoulder lift. Lifting the patient from bed to chair. I.

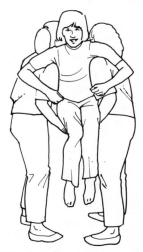

Figure 8.18 Shoulder lift. Lifting the patient from bed to chair. II. The lift. Having lifted the patient from the bed, the lifter's free hand is placed to support the small of the patient's back. When necessary, one lifter can used this free hand to carry an object, such as a tube or an infusion bottle.

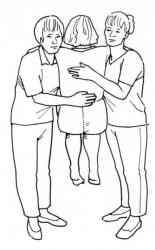

Figure 8.19 Shoulder lift. Lifting the patient from bed to chair. III. After lifting. the lifters turn in an agreed direction to face the chair.

9 Elimination

In everyday life, an adult voids urine, passes faeces and deals with menstrual flow privately, discreetly and in a socially acceptable way. Apart from the more public management of these activities occasioned by living and sleeping in a public ward when in hospital, it may be that disturbances of these functions present medical or nursing problems for the patient. Observation of excreta may form an important part of the evidence leading to diagnosis. For any patient who is physically disabled or bedfast, the problems may become greater since he will have to rely on the nursing staff, relatives, friends, or other carers to cater for these needs.

URINARY FUNCTION

History and assessment of urinary function

In obtaining the nursing history, the following items of information should be included:

1. Whether or not the patient experiences any difficulty or pain in passing urine.
2. A note of the frequency with which urine is normally passed, including any necessity to get out of bed at night in order to void.
3. Whether there is ever any difficulty in detecting the urge to pass urine. Can the patient tolerate an interval

of delay between the first urge to pass urine and the act itself?

4. Any physical disability (including poor vision) which might interfere with the patient using the toilet without help.
5. If the patient is confined to bed, is there likely to be any difficulty in the use of a bedpand?

In assessing the patient, note any incontinence. The first specimen of urine passed by the patient should be retained, observed for colour and smell and tested for abnormalities. If there has been any reduction in the amount of urine passed by the patient, it may be useful to palpate in the suprapubic area (or get the doctor to do this).

The care plan

In writing the care plan, not only should the patient's history and assessment be taken into consideration but also the ward layout. This is particularly important in the case of elderly, infirm patients, who should have their bed or chair sited near to the toilet. The use of the toilet in a mixed ward may be problematic for an elderly patient, where it would be treated casually by a younger one. The signs indicating where the toilet is should be big enough to be read easily and patients should be taken to the toilet for the first time. Any patient who suffers from urgency of micturition or stress incontinence should have this listed as a nursing problem on the care plan. Instructions to offer toilet facilities at regular intervals and immediate response to any request should be stated on the care plan.

The discussion which follows revolves around provision for patients who are confined to bed. A patients who is up in a chair but is relatively immobile has similar problems. Indeed, such a patient's problems may be greater and unless special care is taken incontinence of urine may result.

ADMINISTRATION OF BEDPANS, URINALS AND COMMODES

Bedpans, urinals and commodes should be given as required. Each bed should be screened whilst the patient uses a bedpan or commode, when the patient is in a hospital ward.

Bedpans

These may be made of stainless steel, polypropylene or rubber. They are sterilized after use, by means of a bedpan sterilizer, and are warmed before use either in a heated trolley or by being held under the hot water tap and then thoroughly dried. Nowadays, disposable cardboard bedpans are frequently provided. These are not cold to the skin. They are used once only before disposal in a special machine.

The bedpan is taken to the patient and she is seated comfortably on it, two nurses lifting her if she cannot help herself. She should be supported whilst using the bedpan if she is very weak or ill. When the bedpan is removed it should be covered by a paper cover and may be placed into an unheated trolley. The urine should be measured if the patient is having her fluid intake and output charted, and the amount should be recorded before the urine is emptied and the bedpan washed in the bedpan washer or disposed of. It is then placed into the sterilizer to be sterilized before re-use. The patient is made comfortable and the curtains drawn back.

If the patient has the bowels open, *either* the nurse

should clean the patient using cotton wool swabs, soap and warm water, followed by thorough drying, *or* the patient may be provided with the equipment to carry this out and must be given the opportunity to wash the hands afterwards.

Whenever possible, the patient should be allowed up to the toilet, being taken in a chair and helped by a nurse if necessary. A sanichair, into which a bedpan can be fitted, or a commode, may be used at the bedside, and the patient can be lifted on to it.

Urinals

There is much less formality about the use of urinals, since these can be used unobtrusively under the bed covers, and in general men seem much less self-conscious about passing urine than do women. It is very often the practice for male patients who are confined to bed to have a clean urinal at the bedside, which is emptied after use.

Both bedpans and urinals should be emptied immediately after use to avoid embarrassing patients.

URINARY COMPLICATIONS

In the normal, active, healthy adult, urine is formed continually by the kidney and passes down the ureters to the bladder. The bladder, a hollow muscular organ, fills from its empty, collapsed state until pressure stimulates the stretch receptors in its wall and initiates micturition. This reflex is initiated in the adult when there is a volume of approximately 300 ml of urine within the bladder, but from infancy the act of micturition can be inhibited or facilitated at will. However, this inhibition and facilitation is greatly influenced by emotional factors.

The use of a bedpan or urinal by a patient confined to bed involves passing urine in what is, for persons of our culture, an unnatural position. There are still very few hospitals which supply single rooms for the patients and so, for the vast majority, the voiding of urine is carried out within sound of other patients and hospital staff. Bed curtains ensuring privacy have a disadvantage from the patient's point of view, in that persons wishing to enter the bed space cannot knock before doing so, and therefore do tend to enter without warning. In interviews with patients about the incidents which caused them anxiety and stress in hospital, Wilson-Barnett (1977) found that two-thirds of those interviewed expressed strong feelings against the use of a bedpan. Some would suffer great discomfort waiting to be wheeled to the lavatory rather than use a bedpan. There is a great deal of individual variation in the interval between the urge to pass urine, as well as variation in the tolerance of this urge if it cannot immediately be relieved.

A patient who wishes to micturate and cannot do so immediately may become very anxious and be unable to control the bladder sphincter, wetting the bed as a result. On the other hand, powerful inhibition of the act may mean that he is unable to pass urine when the opportunity to do so does arise. Not all patients, therefore, can regulate their bladders so that they only pass urine at a time dictated by the convenience of the ward staff. This problem is less acute for male patients since there is usually an 'up' patient who is willing to fetch a urinal if asked, and this can be used discreetly. Sensitive female patients may be unwilling to ask an apparently busy nurse for a bedpan because it involves an interruption of whatever task the nurse is carrying out. Indeed, the occasional female patient, confined to bed, finds the whole business such an embarrassment that she will voluntarily restrict her fluid intake so that she will not need to use the bedpan so frequently. This, in a patient lying still in bed, could lead to urinary infection or the formation of renal calculi. Thus the urinary complications of enforced bed rest may be: (1) wetting the bed (a very shameful thing to an adult patient); (2) retention of urine; (3) urinary infection; or (4) renal calculi.

The prevention of urinary complications

One of the most important ways in which a nurse can prevent urinary complications is by developing the capacity to appreciate the patient's embarrassment and fears occasioned by the use of the bedpan. The nurse's attitude toward this problem will be betrayed in her behaviour. She should ensure maximum privacy for the patient and respect that privacy. To reduce embarrassment to a minimum, the nurse should be relaxed and matter of fact when attending to the sanitary needs of the patient. It is essential that the bedpan or urinal should be at a comfortable temperature and scrupulously clean; the nurse must always be willing to supply a bedpan or urinal to the patient when asked, and the patient must be aware of the nurse's willingness in this respect. It is here, particularly, that the nurse's attitude is all important, since verbal willingness accompanied by feeling that the patient is a nuisance may appear false to the patient; facial expression and movements of the body can reveal true attitudes to the onlooker. If possible, the nurse should be sensitive to the facial expressions of patients so that she can anticipate the patient's need to pass urine and offer a receptacle before being asked.

Observation of the urinary output is necessary. This does not necessarily have to be formally charted on a fluid chart, but an assessment of the amount passed and the frequency with which the bedpan or urinal is used can be made in the light of the nurse's experience. The nurse should always bear in mind the possibility that the bladder is not being emptied completely, even though urine is passed; a situation very likely to result in urinary infection. If it is suspected that urine is being retained, then measurement of the patient's fluid intake and output will be necessary and the bladder should be examined to see if it is distended.

Unless the fluid intake is being restricted as part of the treatment, the nurse should ensure that the patient takes sufficient fluid to prevent the complications of infection or calculi from occurring (see Chapter 19).

Observation of the colour, smell and turbidity of the patient's urine should be carried out every time a urinal or bedpan is emptied. If any abnormality is suspected, it should be reported and a specimen should be saved for inspection, so that any urinary infection is detected as soon as it occurs.

The nurse's responsibility if urinary complications should occur

If *urinary infection* is present or suspected, a specimen of urine will be needed for microbiological examination; this must not be contaminated with microorganisms from the container or the external genitalia. The specimen may be collected by means of catheterization but, more usually, a clean midstream specimen of urine is obtained, since there is always a danger of introducing microorganisms into the bladder whenever catheterization is carried out. It may be difficult to obtain a midstream specimen of urine when the patient is confined to bed.

If the patient has *difficulty in passing urine*, attempts may be made to help by using suggestion. Running taps near the patient's bed or, in the case of a female, pouring warm water over the vulva, may initiate the act of micturition. A plain muscle relaxant, such as carbachol (0.2−0.5 mg) may be prescribed by the doctor, but this drug does have unpleasant side-effects (pallor, sweating, defaecation, vomiting and faintness in some patients). If retention of urine develops, then catheterization will be necessary.

Preventing complications when an in-dwelling catheter is used.

If a patient develops retention of urine, the pressure may be relieved gradually, rather than decompressing the bladder suddenly and completely, when the catheter is passed. In either case, it may be necessary to leave the catheter in position and, for this reason, the initial catheterization for retention of urine is often carried out using a self-retaining catheter.

Other reasons for inserting a self-retaining catheter are: (1) to keep the bladder empty during and after gynaecological operations; (2) to ensure careful observation of the urine after operations upon the bladder itself or in its vicinity, and to allow bladder washouts to be carried out if required.

Complications of a self-retaining catheter and their prevention

Inflammation of the urethra may occur as a tissue reaction to the presence of a foreign substance. For this reason the choice of a relatively non-reactive material is recommended in the manufacture of urinary catheters. For short-term use, latex catheters dipped or coated with silicone are used. Another recommendation is the use of Teflon catheters. For long-term catheterization, catheters manufactured from 100% silicone or hydrogel are strongly recommended.

The presence of the catheter lying within the urethra and the bladder sphincter, and so connecting the interior of the bladder to the body exterior, provides a direct pathway into the bladder for microorganisms. Thus, the risk of urinary infection is a very real one when a self-retaining catheter is used, even though the catheterization technique has been carried out safely. Indeed, the danger of infection is such that intermittent catheterization may be preferred over the use of self-retaining catheters for patients who are paraplegic and are unable to pass urine normally.

Usually, a self-retaining catheter is attached via tubing to a drainage bag. The urine may be left to drain freely into the bag or the system may be clamped. In the latter case, the clamp will be opened at prescribed intervals to allow the urine which has accumulated within the bladder to empty. Which of these methods is chosen depends upon the reason for which the self-retaining catheter was inserted in the first place.

Whilst the use of sterile catheter, tubing and drainage bag reduces the possibility of infection, problems may arise once the system has been set up. A major potential problem is that of disconnections of the system. Clearly the system must *never* be disconnected or urinary infection is extremely likely to follow.

The urinary drainage bag should be supported upon a suitable hanger and then placed on the side of the bed or chair in such a way as to allow unobstructed downflow of urine from the bladder. Backflow of urine from the bag or tubing should be avoided, since this allows the migration of microorganisms into the bladder. This position of the bag, below the bladder, must be maintained during bag emptying.

Several precautions should be taken when the bag is emptied. First, the nurse should wash and dry the hands. Contamination of the tap should be avoided during emptying and the tap should be dried thoroughly after it is used. Disposable containers for the collection of the urine are advocated, but in any case both the container and the urine should be disposed of safely. The hands should be washed and dried again at the end of the procedure.

TO COLLECT A MIDSTREAM SPECIMEN OF URINE

Principles

1. Contamination of the urine specimen by organisms from the urethra and genital organs is avoided:
   (a) By thorough cleaning of the urethral orifice and the area around it.
   (b) By allowing any organisms within to be washed away by the first part of the urine stream before the specimen is collected.
2. The cleansing agent used should be mild, to avoid trauma to delicate mucous membranes. If it should contaminate the urine specimen, it should not be strong enough to kill delicate infecting organisms.

Requirements

- Sterile, wide-necked container
- Bedpan or urinal
- Sterile wool or gauze swabs
- Sterile water, or a mild sterile antiseptic lotion, e.g. Hibitane 1:5000
- Normal saline
- Soap and warm water
- Sterile absorbent towels

Procedure (female patient)

The procedure, and the reasons for it, should be explained very carefully to the patient. If possible, the patient should be allowed to carry out the cleaning of the area for herself and an ambulant patient can carry out the whole procedure for herself. The vulva is washed thoroughly with soap and water, using the sterile swabs and working from front to back. The area is thoroughly rinsed with clean water and dried. Next, the area around the urethral orifice is swabbed with the particular lotion in use in the hospital, and dried. The bedpan is placed in position, with the patient leaning forward as far as possible. (An ambulant patient should lean forward on the toilet.) If possible the patient should part the labia minora whilst urine is passed, otherwise the nurse should do this for her. The first part of the urine flow is collected in the bedpan or toilet, then the sterile container is placed in position, the 'midstream' urine is collected, and the bottle is sealed. Any remaining urine is then passed. After the procedure, the patient should be dried thoroughly and made comfortable. The nurse must wash her hands and ensure that the specimen is taken to the laboratory straight away, accompanied by the appropriate request form. Speed is essential or delicate organisms may die whilst less delicate ones multiply, giving a false picture of the infecting agent.

Note. For female ambulant patients the 'Specitest' collector may prove a satisfactory method of collecting a midstream specimen of urine, but it does involve the installation of a special lavatory into the ward.

Procedure (male patient)

Again, a male patient should carry out the procedure for himself as far as is possible, so careful explanation is very important. The penis and especially the area around the urethra should be washed thoroughly with soap and water, rinsed and dried. The prescribed lotion should then be used to cleanse the area immediately around the urethral orifice, the foreskin being pulled back to ensure thorough cleansing. The patient then passes urine into a urinal or toilet before stopping the stream in order to pass the second part of the stream into the sterile container. He must be warned not to let the penis touch the inside of either the urinal or the sterile container.

CATHETERIZATION

Catheterization of the urinary bladder may be required: (1) to empty the bladder before operation; (2) to keep the bladder empty after operation; (3) to obtain a specimen of urine; and (4) to relieve distension.

Principles

1. Precautions are taken to avoid introducing micro-organisms into the urinary system.
2. Trauma of the urethra and bladder is avoided by means of skilful technique, a knowledge of the anatomy of the area, and the use of catheters made of smooth, atraumatic material.

Varieties of catheter in common use

Most varieties of catheter are available in presterilized, individual packs, and are disposable (Figures 9.1–9.3). The central sterile supply department of most hospitals also supplies individually wrapped sterile catheters which are resterilized by them after use. Prepacked catheters are sterilized by gamma rays. The storage of catheters within the ward is important. They should be stored away from heat and sunlight. Before use, the expiry date should be checked.

For female catheterization. Female length catheters should be chosen, of size 10–16 (Charrière). If self-retaining catheters are used they should be made of latex/Teflon, latex/silicone, or 100% silicone. They help to prevent tissue reaction and can be left in place for long periods of time. Balloon sizes should not exceed 5–10 ml.

For male catheterization. For single catheterization, specialized male catheters may be used, but for long-term catheterization self-retaining catheters of male length, made of the materials mentioned above, are used. Again, balloon size should not exceed 5–10 ml. For males with genitourinary problems, larger sizes up to size 26 (Charrière) may be used.

Catheterization of a male patient

Requirements

- The required, prepacked catheters
- Lubricant, such as sterile liquid paraffin, chlorehexidine cream, KY jelly *or* anaesthetic gel

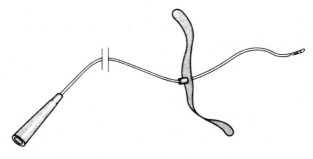

Figure 9.1 Gibbon catheter (male). Note: (1) the end of the catheter has three holes; (2) wings of soft material 30 cm (12 in.) from the catheter tip are secured to the patient's abdomen; (3) a graduated adaptor fits the tube of the collecting bag.

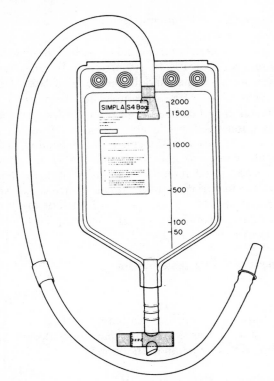

Figure 9.2 Disposable urine collecting and measuring bag for use with indwelling catheters.

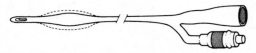

Figure 9.3 Self-retaining Foley catheter.

- Sterile gloves
- Two pairs dissecting, dressing or Spencer Wells forceps
- Container for used instruments
- Disposable bag for dirty dressings
- 1 pair of sterile scissors to cut pack containing catheters
- Sterile towels and swabs
- Bowl of warm lotion for swabbing, e.g. Hibitane 0.1 per cent, Bradosol 1:2000 solution
- Large receiver for urine
- Waterproof sheet
- (If a 'clean' specimen for examination is required, a sterile screw-top bottle to receive the urine must be provided.)

The bed is screened and the bedclothes arranged so that they can be easily turned down over the thighs, leaving the abdomen and chest covered with a blanket.

After the trolley is brought to the bedside the nurse is not usually required to give any further assistance.

If the catheter is to be tied in, the following should also be provided.

- Tape
- Adhesive strapping
- A pair of scissors

Catheterization of a female patient

Requirements

- Prepacked sterile catheter
- Sterile gloves *or* 2 pairs sterile dressing forceps
- Pair of sterile scissors
- Container for used instruments
- Disposable bag for dirty dressings
- Bowl of lotion for swabbing

- Sterile swabs and towels
- Waterproof sheet
- Large receiver for urine (sterile)
- Hand lamp
- Sterile water ⎫
- Syringe   ⎬ If a Foley catheter is to be used
- Adaptor   ⎭
- (When a sterile specimen is required a sterile screw-top bottle should be provided, and all traces of antiseptic should be removed by swabbing with sterile water.)

Lubricant is not as a rule required.

Procedure

The procedure must be explained carefully as it may be very embarrassing. It is important that the patient understands that the urine will flow through the catheter and she need not strain to expel it. She needs reassurance as the procedure progresses as to the purpose of each of the nurse's actions.

1. The bed should be screened and the bedclothes turned down as far as the patient's knees, leaving her covered with a blanket.
2. A waterproof sheet is placed under the patient's thighs and buttocks and a sterile receiver between her legs.
3. The hand lamp should be adjusted so that it gives a good light; it is absolutely essential that the nurse should be able to obtain a clear view of the area when swabbing the external genitalia and when actually passing the catheter. It is a good idea to locate the urethral orifice at this point, before the hands are washed.
4. The nurse then prepares her hands by washing and drying them on a clean towel. The packs of sterile dressings and catheter container are opened and the

contents placed on to the sterile area formed by the inside of the opened out paper towel covering the sterile pack. With her elbow, the nurse turns back the blanket covering the patient, or asks her assistant do this for her.

5. Using swabs well moistened with antiseptic lotion, the nurse swabs the external genital region beginning with the labia majora, then swabbing the labia minora and lastly the area around the urethral orifice. Each swab should be used once only and the direction of swabbing should be from the front of the vulva toward the back.

6. The nurse should then wash her hands and apply sterile gloves if she prefers to handle the catheter with gloves rather than with forceps. In general, the likelihood of contamination is reduced by the use of sterile gloves, as is the possibility of damage to patient tissues, since dexterity and control are so much better.

7. The sterile towels are arranged to cover the patient's thighs and on the mackintosh between the patient's legs, and the sterile receiver is placed on the sterile towel ready to receive the urine.

8. Separating the labia minora, using the first finger and thumb of the left hand, the catheter is passed, using the gloved right hand. (**Note**. Left-handed nurses will obviously use the left hand for passing the catheter.) The urethral orifice should be clearly seen and a good light is essential; the opening is situated immediately in front of the vaginal orifice and at the base of the triangular area known as the vestibule. It is occasionally useful to place a cotton wool swab in the vaginal orifice to help to locate the urethra and to avoid contamination of the sterile catheter by misplacing it into the vagina.

9. The tip of the catheter is passed into the urethral

orifice and then gently pushed in an upward and backward direction for about 5 cm, leaving the open end in the receiver between the patient's thighs. If the catheter should accidentally touch any adjacent part before it is safely inserted into the urethra, it should be discarded and a second sterile catheter used.

10. If a catheter specimen is required for laboratory examination, it is collected in a sterile screw-top glass bottle.

11. When urine ceases to flow the nurse should make gentle pressure over the pubes and withdraw the catheter for about 1 cm; when she feels sure that the bladder is empty the catheter is withdrawn and placed in the receiver provided.

12. The receiver is removed, the vulva dried and the bed remade.

13. The amount of urine withdrawn should be measured and a specimen saved if required.

Catheterization is a procedure that should be carried out with the utmost care, since, by introducing the catheter through the urethra, microorganisms could also be introduced, and the procedure itself may damage the delicate urethral lining.

Catheter toilet

The use of meatal cleansing once a self-retaining catheter is in place may well be recommended in some hospitals or wards. Scientific evidence in relation to this practice is unclear, although it may serve a useful function for aesthetic or comfort reasons.

Principle

An aseptic technique should be used.

Requirements

- Sterile wool or gauze swabs
- Sterile towel
- Sterile water or saline or Hibitaine 1:5000
- Pair of sterile gloves
- Disposal bag for dirty dressings, used gloves

Method

The procedure is explained to the patient and the bed-clothes turned back. The nurse should wash the hands and place the sterile towel in position below the catheter.

After applying the sterile gloves, the nurse swabs the urethral orifice with the prescribed lotion to remove crusts. The exterior of the catheter is also swabbed at its insertion. Dry sterile swabs are used when the cleansing has been completed. Each swab should be used once only and then placed in the disposal bag. Swabbing should be carried out in one direction, i.e. away from the urethral orifice.

URINARY INCONTINENCE

Urinary incontinence has already been mentioned in relation to hospital patients, but it is a much more wide-spread problem than one affecting hospital patients alone. It has been calculated that some three million people in Britain suffer from urinary incontinence (Norton, 1986). The condition occurs more frequently in women than men and is most common in the elderly and the disabled. It is a very disabling condition: the sufferer may be reluctant to go out, self-esteem will suffer, and interpersonal relationships will probably be affected. Apart from these negative effects, considerable expense may be incurred in purchasing suitable pads, undergarments, and additional bed-linen. District health authorities supply incontinence pads to known sufferers but not all sufferers will seek help because of the loss of dignity involved. In any case, due to the purchasing policy imposed upon district health authorities, only a small selection of pad types may be available from this source. Since incontinence can affect individuals of all ages and sizes, the shape, size and absorption qualities of pads need careful matching to individual requirements.

Treatment and management of urinary incontinence is beyond the scope of this book. However, specialist nurse continence advisers provide not only a direct service to individual clients but also an indirect service through their educational/consultancy function. Both district nurses and hospital nurses can seek such advice so that they, in turn, can provide appropriate help to their patients. Continence advisers are not only knowledgeable about the full range of products available to help sufferers to cope with unavoidable incontinence but, above all, can help in the promotion of continence.

BOWEL FUNCTION

When one is healthy, the exercise involved in day-to-day activities helps to maintain the tone of skeletal muscles used in the act of defaecation. Peristalsis is aided by the upright posture in walking or standing, which avoids compression of internal abdominal organs. Most individuals establish very regular bowel habits, involving the use of the lavatory at much the same time each day, often after breakfast. Their diet too, though changing in detail from meal to meal, probably contains fairly constant quantities of dietary fibre, carbohydrate, protein, fat and fluids. When the patient is admitted to hospital, he is denied exercise, his daily routine is modified to suit the hospital, and his diet is changed in both content and timing. All of these factors may cause a change in bowel habit, and usually the change is towards constipation rather than diarrhoea. Given the inhibiting conditions under which a patient confined to bed must defaecate, it is small wonder that constipation is often a problem. Because the use of a bedpan entails an unnatural position and because it has been shown to place a greater strain on the heart than the use of a commode, some physicians allow patients on complete bed rest to be lifted on to a commode. Some of the drugs used in the treatment of the patient can lead to constipation, e.g. morphine and its derivatives. A lot of gas-producing foods in the diet, combined with lack of exercise, may make flatus a real problem too. All of these problems may become more acute after surgery, since peristalsis will have been affected by the anaesthetic during operation, and wound pain may postoperatively seriously impede straining at stool.

A study was carried out by Wright (1974) in which she interviewed 666 patients from eight different hospitals about their bowel function. She found that more women than men and more of the elderly patients than young ones had taken aperients before their admission to hospital.

Sanichairs, although provided in 22 wards, were seldom used. About a half of the patients interviewed had used a bedpan and a third had used the commode. Elderly women patients were the mostly likely to have used the bedpan and male patients to have used a commode, sanichair or to have gone to the toilet by wheelchair. Younger patients were more independent. A bedpan had been used by a high proportion of patients with ischaemic heart disease. (This causes a greater strain on the heart than does using a commode.)

Aperients seemed to be given routinely, prescribed by the ward sister, charge nurse or staff nurse.

Only 29% of patients had been provided with handwashing facilities after using a bedpan or commode to open their bowels.

In the 5 days following admission to hospital, 54.7% of the patients interviewed had less frequent bowel action than at home, and 26.9% had been worried or concerned about their bowels since admission.

Concern was expressed by many patients about using the bedpan; its discomfort, difficulty in use and uncomfortable temperature caused most concern, together with embarrassment. More comments of this kind were received from men than women.

History and assessment of bowel function

Details which will be recorded on the nursing history sheet will include the following.

1. How frequently the patient has a bowel action under normal circumstances.
2. Whether or not the pattern of bowel action has changed during the period before the patient's admission to hospital.
3. If the patient experiences pain or difficulty on defaecation.
4. Whether the patient finds particular foods irritant or predisposing to flatus.
5. Any aperients or laxatives taken at home; their name, the dose taken and the frequency of taking them.
6. Details of the normal diet, activity level, and fluid intake may be important.
7. Any drugs taken which might affect bowel function as a side-effect.

Rather than the nurse carrying out a physical *assessment*, results can be obtained from the doctor, who will carry out rectal examination as part of the admission procedure.

PREVENTION OF BOWEL COMPLICATIONS

In writing the nursing care plan for a patient for whom a potential problem of constipation has been identified, the following points are to be remembered.

1. The diet of the patients is very important and should contain as much fresh fruit and vegetables as possible. Bran may be added to breakfast cereals, the amount being calculated individually for each patient.
2. Doctors and nurses should be aware of the strain that use of the bedpan can put upon the patient, as well as the worry that it may cause. Patients should be allowed to get up to the toilet and use the sanichair as much as possible. A commode is preferable to a bedpan. A request to have the bowels open from a patient must be attended to at once. Privacy must be ensured.
3. Aperients should be prescribed by the doctor for each patient individually and given as prescribed by the nurse.
4. Suppositories or enemata may be administered if constipation does arise. A flatus tube may be passed to relieve wind if this is a problem.
5. Nurses should ensure that they provide hand-washing facilities for the patient after use of the bedpan or commode.
6. Bowel action must be accurately recorded.

Administration of suppositories

Suppositories used to evacuate the bowel are made of glycerine or Dulcolax. Some drugs which can be absorbed through the bowel wall are administered in the form of suppositories. It is important in the latter case that the bowel is empty before the drug is administered and that the reason for the administration of the suppository is carefully explained to the patient so that the suppository is retained.

Requirements

- Prescribed suppositories, together with the prescription sheet
- Rubber gloves *or* two finger stalls
- Petroleum jelly and swab, *or* bowl of hot water
- Waterproof sheet and towel, *or* incontinence pad

Procedure

The waterproof sheet and towel are put in position, to protect the bed, and the patient is positioned, if possible in the left lateral position, with knees and hips well flexed. The procedure should have been very carefully explained to the patient, The gloves or finger stalls are applied and the suppository is lubricated, either by using petroleum jelly or by dipping it into hot water, thus causing the surface to melt slightly. The suppository is inserted through the anal sphincter as far as possible into the rectum. The sheet is removed and the patient is repositioned. An evacuant suppository should be retained about 20 minutes if possible, but the patient may get agitated for fear that the nurse will not get the bedpan or commode to the bedside in time. It is useful to leave one at the bedside to reassure the patient.

Administration of evacuant enemata

Solutions which may be used

- Sodium phosphate disposable enemata
- Water 280–1120 ml
- Soap and water 280–1120 ml

- Magnesium sulphate 25% solution, approximately 224 ml

Principles

1. The patient is positioned so as to take advantage of the natural curvature of the rectum. Therefore, if at all possible, the patient should either lie on the left side or on the back with the pelvis raised slightly.
2. All air must be expelled from the tubing, or it will cause acute discomfort to the patient.
3. The fluid must be measured before and after administration, as it is possible for fluid to be absorbed from the mucous membrane, upsetting the electrolyte balance.
4. The rate of flow of the fluid can be regulated by pinching the tubing with the finger or by altering the height of the funnel above the patient's rectum; the higher it is, the greater the flow rate. The size of the apparatus will also affect the flow rate; thus small, narrow-bore tubing and catheter should be used if only a small amount of fluid is to be administered or if the fluid is to be administered very slowly.

Requirements

- For large quantities of fluid, a douche can, or large funnel, a piece of tubing about 60 cm long, a connector and a rectal tube or catheter size 18−26 (French gauge) or 14−16 (English gauge)
- For small quantities, a glass funnel or the barrel of a glass syringe is connected to a rubber catheter size 12−14 (French gauge) or 8 (English gauge)
- Linen swabs
- Vaseline
- Clip to control the flow of fluid

- Jug containing a measured amount of solution to be administered
- Lotion thermometer
- Disposal bag for soiled equipment
- Bedpan with toilet paper or cheap cotton wool
- Waterproof sheet and protective towel or incontinence sheet

Procedure

It is important that the procedure is explained in terms the patient will understand. The patient is positioned on the waterproof sheet and towel. The temperature of the liquid which is to be administered is checked. This should be at a temperature of 38°C (100°F). Next, the apparatus is filled with fluid, ensuring that there is no air remaining in the tubing, and the tubing is clipped. The catheter is lubricated and gently inserted through the anus into the rectum, until 10 cm have been inserted. In the case of a female patient care should be taken to locate the anus. The catheter must not be forced if there is any resistance, as this may harm the patient. Unscrew the clip on the tubing. Whilst the liquid is running in at the prescribed rate, the nurse must never allow the funnel to become empty of fluid until the completion of the procedure, or air will enter the apparatus. If the patient complains of nausea or faintness at any time, the procedure must be discontinued. The catheter is withdrawn gently and disconnected from the rest of the apparatus so that it can be washed separately. The patient is placed on to the bedpan or commode, and supported if necessary. On emptying the bedpan, the fluid must be measured to ensure that the whole amount administered has been returned. Careful observation and reporting of the faecal and flatus result of the enema should be carried out.

Passing a flatus tube for the relief of distension

Requirements

- Rubber rectal tube. This tube has thick walls and the eye is at the end. (In this respect it differs from a catheter, which has a lateral eye.) A connector attaching the rectal tube to a length of tubing with a funnel at the other end
- Petroleum jelly, or other lubricant and swabs
- Bowl of water
- Receiver for soiled swabs
- Waterproof square and pad to protect the bed
- Plastic disposable gloves

The tube is lubricated and passed into the rectum to a depth of about 5 cm. The funnel is placed under the surface of the water in the bowl which is placed at the bedside. The advantage of attaching the tube to a funnel placed in a bowl of water is that the bubbles of gas can be readily seen as they escape from the funnel.

Evacuant suppositories may also be administered to relieve flatus.

10 Providing for patient hygiene and comfort: the patient and the self-image

In normal adult life, bathing, washing, tooth cleaning, etc. (activities of daily living) are important but unproblematic. They become routine activities, frequently carried out in complete privacy or at the most, in the presence only of the immediate nuclear family.

When a person is ill or disabled it may become difficult to carry out these activities of daily living. We have probably all experienced the problems which arise if just one hand is out of action for a trivial reason, such as a cut. Nurses need to know how people can be helped to cope. For example, by wrapping a plastic bag around an injured extremity and showering rather than bathing.

It may be necessary for these basic activities to be carried out for a patient by someone else. This raises the following issues.

1. Issues of self-esteem, since being washed or bathed by someone else usually only occurs in infancy.
2. Issues of privacy will be important for the elderly in particular. It may be that throughout their lives few people, with the exception of the spouse, have been allowed to see the person naked.
3. Issues relevant to the self-image and presentation of the self. When someone else is responsible for a person's hygiene the standard achieved may be less than

their normal standard. The application of make-up or achieving a particular hair style may become problematic when someone else is doing this for the patient.

BODY IMAGE CHANGE

Bathing, in particular, may cause great anxiety to a patient whose condition involves body image change. Bathing carried out by a nurse may be the very first occasion on which a patient is testing another's reaction to body image change. The way in which the nurse handles the situation is absolutely crucial to the way in which the patient will come to terms with what has happened.

Body image has been defined by Norris (1970) as 'the constantly changing total of conscious and unconscious information, feeling and perceptions about ones body in space as different and apart from all others ... It is basic to identity'. There is very close interdependence between body image, personality, ego, self-image and identity. Body image changes occur throughout the normal healthy life span, especially at puberty, in pregnancy, childbirth and the menopause. Corbeil (1971) argued that body image change may be related more to perceived bodily change than to actual body change. Change in body image probably occurs every time one is ill, injured or disabled. None the less, some conditions involving body image change have a greater impact upon patients than others. The rapidity of the change, its permanence and its visibility are all factors which influence the magnitude of impact. Conditions such as mastectomy, limb amputation, severe burns, cancer and stoma formation are ones in which the body image change is a very important consideration. Responses to body image change include anxiety, depression, shame, hopelessness and fear. The patient needs to work through a process of adaptation to the changed body image. This can be helped by beginning the process preoperatively in a patient undergoing a planned operation.

Roberts (1976) described the following stages in the process of adaptation to changed body image.

1. *Impact*. This occurs at the time of the physical change and is manifest by numbness, dissociation, despair and depression. Extreme passivity can occur.
2. *Retreat*. Here the person begins to handle the impact psychologically. Threat is felt and denial may occur. The future is perceived as very bleak.
3. *Acknowledgement*. During this phase the individual either mentally, or in overt discussion, goes over the events which lead to the physical change, attempting to make sense of what has happened. There may be an attempt to find cause—effect relationships which did not actually occur. Self-esteem may be very low, with uncertainty about the future.
4. *Reconstruction*. This is the point at which the individual comes to terms with the change and faces the future.

It is important to realize, that, as with so many processes which are described in stages, any one patient may fail to show this orderly progression. Stages may fail to occur, the order may change and, indeed, the patient may show great lability, rapidly changing from one type of reaction to another. Descriptions such as the one above are conceptual aids to our understanding.

The nursing role

The nurse can do little to help actively, at least as far as our present state of knowledge is concerned.

Assessment is important to identify the patient's perception of what has happened. It may be necessary for the nurse to define to the patient what has occurred. The patient must be allowed both time and privacy to mourn and to grieve for the loss of the old body image. As adaptation begins, the situation can be discussed with the patient, identifying their coping strengths and assets. The patient should be encouraged to look at the physical effects of injury, disease or operation in privacy and to touch the area as soon as it is possible. This helps the changed part to be incorporated into the new body image.

Support of family and friends is important. Clearly, the reactions of staff and family to the physical change is crucially important to the patient. Any negative reaction may create a stigma and prolong the adaptation period.

Bathing is an opportunity for the patient to test out the staff members' reactions but is also an opportunity for staff to begin to get the patient inspecting the wound or damaged area and then later to touch it.

PATIENT HYGIENE

Maintenance of the general cleanliness of a patient in terms of skin, mouth and hair is important for several reasons. Firstly, from the point of view of preventing cross-infection or infection of the patient, who is rendered more vulnerable through illness. A second reason, which cannot be overemphasized, is to contribute to the maintenance of the patient's comfort and self-esteem. The majority of people in the UK value personal cleanliness and use deodorants and perfumes freely as an important aspect of the way in which they present themselves to others. Any lowering of standards of appearance whilst in hospital may cause embarrassment or even severe depression in a person who sets great store by personal appearance.

It is far more difficult to plan care for the minority of people who normally prefer not to wash frequently. Their needs for normal routine have to be weighed against the possible risk of cross-infection to others and the negative attitudes other patients and some staff might display toward them, and advice may need to take this into account.

History and assessment

Details recorded will include the following:

1. The patient's normal frequency of bathing and preference for the use of bathtub or shower.
2. Any problems of mobility likely to interfere with bathing.
3. Note should be made of the patient's preferred hairstyle so that the hair can be dressed during any period of helplessness or coma.
4. The state of the natural teeth and the presence of any dentures or plates should be noted.
5. Times at which the patient normally cleans the teeth should be recorded.

In planning care it is normal to make provision for daily bathing and more frequent washes of face and hands. Frequency of mouth toilet will be mentioned later. Patients who are mobile should be shown the way to the bathroom or shower on admission.

BATHING PATIENTS

If it is at all possible, the patient should bath in the bathroom, or better still, use a shower if one is avaiable, rather than have a bed bath. Practically any patient who can sit out of bed for long periods can be lifted into a bath, or can sit in a special chair whilst being given a shower.

Procedure for bathing a patient in the bathroom

1. Ensure that the air temperature in the bathroom is warm and that the bath has been cleaned and disinfected after the last patient. Take the patient's washing equipment and towels to the bathroom together with clean pyjamas or nightdress and place on the towel rail to warm.

2. Fill the bath with water at a suitable temperature, e.g. 38°C. If the patient is to be lifted into the bath, only about 20 cm of water should be drawn before he is lifted in.

3. *If the patient can bath independently*, leave him whilst bathing. Since most ward bathroom doors have no lock, a screen can be placed around the bath to give a degree of privacy.

4. *If the patient is to be lifted into the bath*, it is useful to place the wheelchair at the end of the bath, opposite the taps, with the patient facing in the direction he will sit in the bath. At least two nurses will be needed to lift the patient on to the edge of the bath; from there he can be gently lowered into the water.

5. Add more water, taking care not to scald the patient with water from the hot water tap (a mixer tap is best), and wash the patient thoroughly. Parts of the body not in the water should be rinsed and dried immediately.

6. The water should then be let out of the bath, and the patient dried as much as possible before being lifted back into the chair.

7. A clean, dry, warm towel, should be placed in the chair to dry the buttocks. Again, the patient can be lifted in two stages, first to the edge of the bath and

then to the chair. He is then dried thoroughly, talcum powder applied, and clean pyjamas, slippers and dressing gown are replaced.

It is possible to get special bath lifts and hoists which are useful to help lift a heavy patient in and out of a bath.

Bathing a patient in bed

Principles

1. Unless a patient is very ill, it is better if he can be bathed daily.
2. Ensure the comfort of the patient throughout the procedure. Carry out as much of the bath as possible before moving the patient from the original comfortable position. Carefully arrange the procedure so that the minimum of movement and turning is required. Rinse and dry the washed areas thoroughly; do not wet such a large area that the patient gets cold and uncomfortable before being dried. Keep the patient warm throughout the procedure.
3. Let the patient carry out as much of the bath for himself as possible. It may be neccessary to hand the flannel and towel. If possible, place the bowl of water on a towel, on the bed, so he can place his hands and feet into it, to soak and wash them.
4. Change the water as often as necessary so that it remains warm and clean, and always change it immediately after washing the pubic area. The water should be as hot as the nurse can tolerate, because considerable cooling of the water on the flannel will occur before it reaches the patient's skin.
5. Make sure that everything needed for the bath is at the bedside before beginning so that the patient is not left during the procedure.

6. The patient should feel refreshed as well as being clean at the end of the bath. Mouth care should be given, nails should be clean and smooth, talcum powder and/or deodorant should be applied; the patient's hair should be brushed, and in the case of a woman, make-up should be applied if she normally wears it. For patients who have been in hospital for a long time, a visit from a beautician can be of great benefit to morale. Similarly the use of a depilatory should be considered, particularly for elderly ladies. If the patient has been unable to take a bath for some time before coming into hospital, special attention should be paid to the cleanliness of the umbilicus and toes.

Requirements

Equipment should preferably be placed on a trolley, which can then act as a working surface and is better than using the top of the patient's locker.

- Clean bed-linen, nightdress or pyjamas
- Container for dirty linen
- Bowl containing hot water
- Jugs containing fresh hot water
- Lotion or bath thermometer
- Bath blankets
- Tooth mug and receiver or mouth tray
- Nail file, hair brush and comb
- Flannels, soap and towels for face and body
- Talcum powder
- Bucket for dirty water

Method

1. Explain the procedure to the patient and offer the opportunity to pass urine. Screen the bed.

2. Strip the top bedclothes, leaving the patient covered with a bath blanket, and one of the blankets from the bed as well if the day is cold. The bath blanket can be put in position simultaneously with the removal of the sheet so that the patient is never completely uncovered. Place the second bath blanket in position underneath the patient by rolling him from side to side.

3. Remove the patient's nightdress or pyjamas.

4. Wash, rinse and dry the face, or better still, allow the patient to do this. Only use soap if this is the normal practice for the patient.

5. Wash, rinse and dry the arm furthest away from you. (This is useful if another nurse is helping; she can then dry the limb whilst the one nearer to you is washed.)

6. Wash, rinse and dry the other arm, the chest, the abdomen and the legs, making sure that the bath blanket covers the parts not actually being washed.

7. The pubic area may be washed next; if the patient can manage this, the nurse can hold the bath blanket up as a 'tent' so the patient has room to work without being embarrassingly exposed. If the patient cannot manage alone, the nurse must give the area a thorough wash.

8. Remove all the pillows except one, and roll the patient on to the side to face away from the nurse who is washing, the second nurse providing support. Using clean water, wash the upper part of the back, then the buttocks, anal region, and pubic area if this has not already been done. Treat the pressure areas and make this side of the bed.

9. Roll the bath blanket to the middle.

10. Turn the patient to the other side, wash and treat pressure areas as necessary. Attend to the bottom

sheets and remove the bath blanket from underneath.
11. Put on clean pyjamas, position the patient comfortably, and remake the bed. Attention to mouth toilet, nails and hair can then be given.

To wash the patient's back. If the patient cannot lie flat or prefers to sit up, support him sitting forward, so the back is exposed, and can be washed and dried. Put on the pyjama jacket. Attend to the bedclothes at the head of the bed whilst the patient is leaning forward, rolling in clean linen as necessary. Replace the pillows and allow the patient to lean back. One nurse can then support the patient's buttocks free of the bed, whilst the other washes the area, carries out pressure area care, and makes the bottom of the bed.

CARE OF THE PATIENT'S HAIR

The patient's hair should be brushed and combed and put into the usual style each morning if the patient is unable to do this unaided. Any patient who is in hospital for a long time may need the hair washing and the nurse must be able to do this, although many hospitals have a hairdresser who visits the ward at regular intervals, and will wash and set the patient's hair.

CARE OF THE MOUTH

Epithelial tissues line the mouth and cover the tongue, and the upper layers keratinize. Friction from the muscular movement involved in eating and talking aids normal desquamation of the keratinized layer, and the saliva then helps to wash the shed cells away. Saliva also dilutes and washes away microorganisms, as well as having a mildly antiseptic action. Any condition, then, which reduces either the normal muscular activity of mouth structures, or the amount of saliva present, will predispose to mouth infection. Worse still, the presence of any instrument or appliance in the mouth can lead to a tissue reaction, or may allow the accumulation of debris. An airway, a Ryle's or oesophageal tube, dentures or an endotracheal tube all increase the risk of damage or infection of the membranes with which they are in contact.

Conditions which reduce the quantity of saliva are as follows.

1. Dehydration due to insufficient fluid intake or to excess sweating, as in fever.
2. Mouth breathing.
3. Lack of reflex stimulation of salivary glands by food, e.g. when the patient is being fed artificially.
4. Administration of drugs which dry salivary secretions, e.g. atropine, scopolamine, antihistamines.
5. In anxiety, when the sympathetic nervous system is overactive.

Lack of normal mouth hygiene leads to halitosis, collection of dried secretion, microorganisms and shed cells, and eventually to mouth infection. Infection can then spread to nasal structures, or the respiratory tract. Conversely, a pre-existent infection of nasal structures or respiratory tract will predispose to mouth infection. The importance of mouth hygiene in sick people cannot be overemphasized and, where the patient cannot undertake this for himself, the nurse must assess the best method and the frequency of mouth care.

For the patient who is not seriously ill, the best method of caring for the mouth is by cleaning the teeth and the tongue, using a soft toothbrush and toothpaste. This removes debris and stimulates the blood supply, maintaining the gums in a healthy condition. An antiseptic mouthwash may be pleasant for the patient, but it is no substitute for cleaning the teeth, and it should be very mild or it will irritate the oral tissues.

When the patient is too ill to clean the teeth, or for the nurse to do it for him, then the nurse must clean the mouth using swabs and lotions.

Assessment of the frequency of mouth care and the method of choice

1. Use the nursing history to check how frequently the patient normally cleans his own teeth. if his mouth is clean, moist and fresh smelling, the normal routine is obviously satisfactory.
2. Check the factors mentioned above as instrumental in reducing the quantity of saliva, e.g. any dehydration, artificial feeding, administration of any drugs which dry secretions, anxiety. If any of these factors are present, more frequent mouth care is necessary, and if possible the fluid intake should be increased.
3. Inspect the mouth and tongue, noting any deterioration of the mucous membrane, tooth infection and the presence of dried secretions or halitosis. Any of these factors will indicate that frequent mouth care is necess-ary. This may be as frequent as 2-hourly or even hourly. The objective of care will be to maintain healthy moist membranes and a fresh-smelling mouth.
4. The method used will depend upon the patient's level of mobility and activity.

If a patient is able to sit up in bed to clean the teeth, he should be supported in a comfortable position with a towel to protect the jacket and the sheet. A tooth glass or metal mug containing tepid or hot water according to preference, toothpaste, brush and a large receiver or basin are required. If the patient cannot sit up, he should be turned to the left side with the towel spread under the head and neck, and the receiver on the towel, conveniently placed to spit into.

A patient who is not able to assist himself should lie on the side. The teeth are cleaned by brushing systematically with a moist toothbrush and the dentifrice, beginning with the outer surfaces of the front teeth, then with the patient opening the mouth wide enough to allow the brush to be inserted between the inner surface of the cheek and the teeth; clean first the teeth on the right side and then on the left side and finally brush the inner surface of the teeth. The teeth should be brushed by starting at the gum margin and working towards the edge of the tooth. The patient should be allowed to rinse freely during the process and, if he cannot raise the head sufficiently to use a tooth glass, an angled drinking tube should be provided. The state of the tongue and mouth should be noted during the tooth-cleaning process. False teeth must receive frequent attention; they should be scrubbed in clean warm water with a small brush, using bicarbonate of soda or a special dentifrice. The patient should be given a mouth wash after the dentures have been cleaned and replaced.

If the patient possesses an electric toothbrush, this may prove a very effective method of keeping teeth and mouth in good condition.

Cleaning the mouth of an ill patient

The aim of cleaning the mouth of an ill patient is to maintain the mouth in a normal condition, i.e. with moist tongue, lips and mucous membranes free from sores and odour, and with teeth clean. If this condition is not maintained, the procedure must be carried out with greater frequency.

Principles

1. Dried secretions, keratinized cells, and microorganisms

are loosened and removed from the epithelial surface by the use of swabs soaked in sodium bicarbonate or hydrogen peroxide solutions.

2. A mildly antiseptic mouthwash solution is used to freshen the mouth.

3. The salivary glands are stimulated by the action of swabbing the mouth. Occasionally lemon juice may be given for the patient to sip to increase the amount of salivary secretion.

4. Dry, cracked lips may easily become infected and this infection could spread to the mouth. Petroleum jelly or the patient's own face cream applied to the lips will prevent the skin from cracking.

5. If herpes simplex lesions are present on the lips, they should be treated by applying an appropriate antiseptic lotion, preventing the spread of this virus.

6. Great care should be taken when cleaning the mouth of an unconscious patient that neither lotion nor a piece of swab is allowed to enter the nasopharynx, from whence it could enter the respiratory system. The use of hydrogen peroxide which froths, cotton wool and gauze from which small pieces may fray should be avoided. Stitched gauze strips, firmly clipped into artery forceps should be used instead (Figure 10.1).

7. The mouth should be cleaned frequently enough to keep the membranes pink and moist, and the breath odourless.

8. Disposable gloves should be used to protect the nurse's hands.

Requirements

- Small bowl containing linen swabs or gauze strips
- Pair of artery forceps and a pair of dissecting forceps
- Gallipots containing hydrogen peroxide, 2.5 volumes *or* sodium bicarbonate, 1:60 solution; glycothymoline

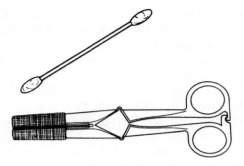

Figure 10.1 'Cotton buds' or Spencer Wells forceps with stitched gauze strip applied may be used for mouth care.

or some other suitable antiseptic solution; glycerine, lemon or glycerine and borax; petroleum jelly
- Disposal bag for soiled swabs
- A bag for soiled forceps
- Towel to protect the patient's chest or bedclothes
- Disposable plastic gloves

Artery forceps and gauze may be replaced with commercially made cotton buds.

Method

Secure the linen or gauze swabs in the forceps so that the ends of the forceps are completely protected by the swab. Moisten them with the hydrogen peroxide or sodium bicarbonate solution and gently swab the epithelial surfaces of the mouth and the surfaces of the teeth. Use the swabs once only, removing the dirty swabs from the forceps by means of the dissecting forceps. Swab the area again using the antiseptic lotion. Glycerine and borax, glycerine or lemon can then be applied, if desired.

Finally, apply petroleum jelly or cream to the lips by means of a swab held in the fingers.

11 Activity and prevention of complications due to inactivity and immobility

It is probable that people have never before had as much opportunity to be sedentary as is possible in today's 'developed' societies. This has led to the recognition of the ill-effects of sedentary life-styles. Exercise, activity and mobility are necessary for satisfactory physiological function and therefore for health.

A brief outline of the physiological effects of exercise and activity on the major systems of the body will follow, together with a short account of the effects of disuse of these systems.

Musculature and bone

During exercise, nerve impulses initiate motor end-plate potentials through the release of acetylcholine. This chemical transmitter is rapidly destroyed by the enzyme cholinesterase. Regular exercise has the effect of increasing the ability of the nerve to manufacture, store and release acetylcholine. Cholinesterase production is also increased. The blood vessels supplying muscles dilate during exercise, and with regular exercise those muscle groups affected increase in bulk and strength. Exercise ensures that muscles are regularly pulling upon bone.

Disuse of muscle leads to weakness and loss of bulk.

There is reduced ability to produce acetylcholine, the speed of its release is slowed and the amount of cholinesterase is reduced. Prolonged inactivity of muscle, with the consequent reduced pull on bone, can lead to the decalcification of bone. This effect is clearly to be avoided in individuals at risk of osteoporosis.

Circulatory system

During exercise, the heart rate and stroke volume increase, leading to an increased cardiac output of blood in unit time. However, since the blood vessels supplying muscles are dilated (see above), as are cutaneous blood vessels, there is at most only a very slight rise in systolic blood pressure, whilst, if anything, the diastolic pressure may fall slightly. In the individual taking regular exercise the resting heart rate and blood pressure tend to fall.

During exercise there is a great increase in the venous return to the heart due to the pumping action of the calf muscles (known as the muscle pump) and the sucking action of the respirations which are greatly increased in depth (known as the thoracic pump). Blood from the viscera is mobilized. Thus, there is no stagnation or pooling of blood.

After periods of time with lack of exercise, the heart rate increases in response to relatively small amounts of additional demand due to low grade exercise. During immobility, especially whilst lying flat (e.g. to ensure spinal column immobility), the cardiac reflexes become sluggish, especially the baroreceptors which adjust the blood pressure to the head and brain. Consequently the individual may faint on sitting up or standing.

Sudden exercise following relative immobility may be dangerous for individuals with coronary heart disease. The sudden demand made on the heart increases the demand on coronary vessels and they may be unable to meet it, resulting in myocardial infarction.

Respiration

During exercise there is increased ventilation of the lungs. Both the diaphragm and the intercostal muscles are active and all the alveoli fill with air. At the same time there is an increase in pulmonary blood flow, with good perfusion of alveoli allowing efficient gas exchange. In regular exercise the whole respiratory system becomes more efficient and the period of oxygen debt after exercise becomes shortened.

In prolonged inactivity the tidal volume of the lungs becomes reduced, leading to poor aeration of alveoli. Some become disused, stagnate and at risk from infection.

Alimentary system

Exercise aids peristalsis and also tones the muscles associated with defaecation (e.g. diaphragm and abdominal muscles).

Constipation may be a side-effect of prolonged inactivity.

Exercise

Clearly the type and amount of exercise taken depends upon the individual's preference, age and the time they have available. Sport is popular, since this has social and other enjoyable features associated with it. Many people take time each day to run or jog, although this may be difficult for those living in cities or other places without access to suitable traffic-free areas. It can also be difficult for full-time workers in the winter, when it is dark by the time one gets home in the evening. Nowadays, walking at a relatively fast pace is considered as good as jogging. It is worth considering the possibility of walking to work, to the station, to the shops, instead of using the bus or car. Swimming is also considered to be an excellent form of exercise. Whatever form of exercise is carried out, it is important that it should be regular, for example, at least twice a week.

In advising people about exercise it is worth identifying a form of exercise they will enjoy. This is especially true for elderly people. For example, dancing is an excellent form of exercise and one which may be enjoyed particularly by elderly people, since it gets them out and interacting with others.

PROBLEMS ASSOCIATED WITH BED REST

A healthy person is ever active. Humans constantly change their position in small ways, even when apparently sitting or standing still. Constant activity is necessary to maintain an adequate blood supply to all tissues. Deprived of blood, tissue cells die, the length of survival depending upon the particular type of cell and its activity level. The movement necessary to maintain the circulation is witnessed by the occasional fainting of healthy young guardsmen standing absolutely still on parade.

In hospital, a patient is encouraged to be as active as possible, but may be incapable of changing position unaided; activity may cause pain, or being active may conflict with a specific need for rest as part of treatment. Good nursing care ensures that the patient will not develop complications due to inactivity, which would delay return to health.

Complications likely to develop as a result of inactivity in bed are beds sores, deep vein thrombosis, urinary complications, and constipation.

PREVENTION OF PRESSURE SORES

Pressure sores are caused by constant pressure on small blood vessels supplying the skin, which reduces the blood flow to the area and prevents the epithelial cells from obtaining the glucose and oxygen they need to maintain life. Soft tissue becomes compressed between the weight of the body, which is transmitted through bone, and the surface of the bed or chair supporting the body. This occurs especially where there is very little protective tissue other than skin between bone and support surface. Small blood vessels become distorted and tear, causing small haemorrhages and depriving the tissue of its blood supply. Pressure sores may also be caused by a shearing force, when the patient sits up in bed. Cohesive forces between skin and sheet may cause stress forces within tissues; surfaces slide over one another, injuring blood vessels. The load of pressure on the tissue is greatly increased (Scales, 1975). Epithelial cells die and the skin breaks, leaving an area of raw tissue. New cells must be formed by division of existing cells, to replace the dead tissue. For this, a good blood supply is essential. Microorganisms can enter an area where the protective integrity of the skin is lost. They readily multiply in such an area, which provides ideal conditions for their growth (warmth, moisture and nutrients). The defences of the body against microorganisms (antibodies, macrophages, white blood cells) are for the most part derived from the blood. Thus a good blood supply is necessary to combat infection, and poor blood supply not only causes the sore but prevents it from healing when it occurs.

Once a pressure sore has developed it may deteriorate very rapidly, due both to infection and the further death of cells; the sore increasing in area and depth. A deep, so-called type II sore is the most difficult to heal. Eventually bone may be exposed, grafting is required to cover the area, and the patient is seriously ill. It can be seen how essential it is that pressure does not build up for a sufficient length of time to interfere with the blood supply to an area of skin.

The responsibilities of the nurse

Prevention of pressure sores is the responsibility of the nurse, and involves the assessment of both the type of care most suitable for the patient and the frequency with which it needs to be carried out. For this it is necessary to have a thorough knowledge of the factors predisposing to pressure sores and of the areas most subjected to pressure in different positions. Other factors which must be taken into account in deciding the particular measures necessary are the activity level of the patient and the nutritional state of the tissue.

Factors which predispose to pressure sores

There are various factors, both intrinsic to the patient and extrinsic, which increase the individual's vulnerability to pressure sores.

Intrinsic factors

Intrinsic factors rendering a person more susceptible to pressure include low activity levels, poor nutritional status, poor physical state and immobility. The ageing process leads to reduced elasticity and increased dryness of the skin, loss of muscle bulk and loss of subcutaneous fat. It is not therefore surprising that vulnerability to pressure increases in the very elderly.

Extrinsic factors

Extrinsic factors include circumstances affecting the micro-environment of the skin subjected to pressure. Dampness (humidity), change in pH and increased temperature are the main factors increasing the likelihood of skin breakdown. Clearly, an existing skin break in an area subjected to pressure also greatly increases the probability of a sore occurring.

Several risk-estimating tools have been devised to determine an individual's degree of vulnerability to pressure sores. These risk estimates incorporate many of the intrinsic and extrinsic factors mentioned above. The Norton scale (Norton et al, 1962) is one of the most simple of these and by far the most popular. Luckily it is as efficient in estimating risk as the other methods.

The Norton scale. This is a simple and reliable way of evaluating a patient's general condition and his liability to develop pressure sores. A patient is assessed on each of five variables and can score from one to four on each of those variables (Table 11.1). Scores are then added. The lower the patient's total score the greater the risk that he will develop a sore: any patient with a score lower than 14 is at risk, whilst a score lower than 12 indicates a particularly worrying level of risk.

Using the scoring system, the frequency of attention to

Table 11.1   The Norton scoring system.

Physical condition		Mental condition		Activity		Mobility		Incontinence	
Good	4	Alert	4	Ambulant	4	Full	4	None	4
Fair	3	Apathetic	3	Able to walk with help	3	Slightly limited	3	Occasionally	3
Poor	2	Confused	2	Chairbound	2	Very limited	2	Usually/ urine	2
Very bad	1	In a stupor	1	Confined to bed	1	Immobile	1	Doubly	1

pressure areas for any individual patient can be determined.

Undergoing a general anaesthetic and surgery

Natural protective reflexes are lost under general anaesthetic unless the procedure is very brief and the anaesthetic light. In deep coma, small movements, including reflexes maintaining muscle tone, are lost. During operation the blood pressure may fall, reducing the blood supply to the skin. The surfaces on which the patient's body rests are frequently hard (e.g. trolleys and operating theatre tables), and, of necessity, the position remains unchanged for the duration of a lengthy operation.

All these factors increase the risk of pressure sores occurring, but when the patients undergoing such procedures are particularly vulnerable, through age, for example, the risk becomes very great indeed.

One condition in which the incidence of pressure sores is high is fractured neck of femur (Royal College of Physicians, 1989) which is most frequently due to osteoporosis in the UK. Osteoporosis affects very elderly people, and women more than men. Not only do these very old people have their fracture attended to under general anaesthetic but they may also have been resting on a hard stretcher/trolley for some time when first admitted to hospital.

Areas at special risk

Skin areas particularly subjected to pressure when the patient is lying supine are the heels, the area overlying the sacrum, the skin over the shoulder blades, the back of the head and the elbows. The sacrum and heels are also subjected to considerable pressure when the patient is in the sitting position. In the lateral and semi-prone positions, the tips of the shoulder, the hips, the inner aspect of the knees, and the ankles are the areas most at risk. Careful placing of sorbo pads or pillows and the use of a bed cradle can prevent pressure on knees and ankles. The areas of skin over the anterior superior iliac spines and over the knees need careful inspection when the patient has been lying in the prone position.

Methods by which pressure may be relieved

Since pressure sores develop as a result of the body weight being transmitted through a fairly small area of tissue, it follows that the smaller the area through which such weight is transmitted the greater the risk of tissue breakdown. Thus, hard ridges in the surfaces on which the body rests, due to creases in the sheets or night clothes, crumbs, etc., greatly increase the risk of sores. Similarly, the harder the surface on which the body rests, the greater the potential for damage. Therefore, patients should not be left for long periods sitting on metal bedpans or commodes, or lying on trolleys in Accident and Emergency or X-ray departments.

On the other hand, most methods of preventing pressure sores rely on relieving the pressure on a particular area, redistributing the pressure from one area to another or spreading the pressure over a larger surface area.

Frequent changes of the patient's position

The greater the number of different positions which are available for use, the better, since pressure on a given area will be relieved for longer if, say, four positions can be used in rotation than if only two positions are used alternately. Frequency of the position changes needs to be determined individually for each patient, and depends both upon any predisposing factors which may be present and the activity level of the patient, but in any case it should not be less than 4-hourly during the daytime. If signs of pressure are noted when the patient is turned, this means that the patient's needs have not been accurately assessed and more frequent attention must be instituted.

The first sign of pressure is redness of an area of skin on which the patient has been lying. If this redness does not disappear rapidly when the patient is turned, then tissue damage has already occurred and the area must be given time to recover before the patient is allowed to lie on it again. The first symptom of pressure is numbness. Patients should be asked to report numbness so that they can be moved immediately it occurs.

Momentary relief of pressure

The patient's condition may be such that he must be nursed in one particular position and it is not possible to turn him. Pressure may be relieved by lifting him up from the surface of the bed for a second. This must be carried out very frequently, even half hourly.

Use of pressure redistributing devices

Several commercial products are available to help to relieve pressure upon an area of tissue; however, good maintenance and a thorough knowledge of the optimum conditions for the use of these is needed or they will do more harm than good. Since many of these aids are expensive, careful assessment is necessary to ensure that the patient will benefit from the use of a particular type of aid.

Gel or foam pads and cushions may be provided to protect a particularly vulnerable area of tissue such as the sacrum, heels or elbow.

Sheepskin bootees are also useful to protect heels and ankles. A large sheepskin may be placed under a patient's sacral area/hips. Frequently, artificial sheepskins are used rather than natural ones because they are more easily laundered.

Special mattresses may be used for patients at high risk of developing sores. They are also used for patients with an established sore,

Ripple beds of two different types are manufactured; large cell and small cell. These consists of a double layer of plastic sealed into long cells (rather like a duvet). A first set of altenate cells is inflated by an electric air pump, whilst the second set is deflated. About 6 minutes later the first set is deflated and the second set inflated. This cycle is constantly repeated. Thus, the pressure is automatically redistributed at frequent intervals. One sheet only must be used between the mattress and the patient, or the bed's efficiency is reduced.

The Pegasus air wave bed consists of two ripple mattresses placed on top of one another. Fleece is used over the top surface of the top mattress. The bed is aerated by a pump, which inflates and deflates the cells.

A water bed is particularly useful for preventing sores in unconscious patients. When used for conscious patients it can be disorienting and they may also find spontaneous movement difficult. This, in turn, may create additional problems. Lifting or moving the patient on these beds is difficult; overhead hoists are provided to help. Careful monitoring is needed to ensure that the thermostat is maintaining the correct water temperature and that there are no leaks.

It is important to remember that these appliances are aids only, and not substitutes for frequent changes of position.

Treatment of a pressure sore

Good nursing care will ensure that pressure sores do not occur. If one should develop, it is treated in the same way as any other wound. Infection is treated, dead tissue is removed using an aseptic technque, and sterile dressings are used to cover the area. Under no circumstances should the patient be allowed to lie on the broken area. Ultraviolet light locally and a high protein diet may be ordered to aid regeneration.

DEEP VEIN THROMBOSIS

One very important protective mechanism of the body is the ability of the blood to clot, given certain conditions which are present in injury. Along with that ability other mechanisms have, however, evolved, which prevent the blood from clotting within the blood vessels themselves. These mechanisms include the property of the platelets to repel each other, thus preventing large aggregates of solid material. Certain substances essential for the clotting process are contained within platelets and tissue cells, and only become available in quantity when there is damage to these cells. The smooth endothelial lining prevents particles from adhering to it, and the flow of blood in the vessels is such that under normal circumstances the larger solid particles tend to remain in the centre of the stream. In addition, small amounts of heparin (an anti-clotting agent) are carried in the bloodstream.

However, given changes in the equilibrium between the anticoagulant and the clotting mechanism, it is possible for blood to clot within the blood vessels. When an individual remains still in bed for a period of time, changes may occur in blood flow and the lining of the veins of the lower limb.

Blood flow in the veins of the lower limb is aided by the pumping action of the calf muscles on movement, and the sucking action of the changes in pressure in the inferior vena cava, consequent upon breathing. Inactivity in bed results in a slowing of the blood flow from the lower limbs, since not only are the calf muscles less active but respiration may be less deep than normal. In the supine or sitting position the veins may become compressed between the bed and the bones of the lower limb; this further slows the circulation and may damage the delicate lining of the vessel. Solid particles of the blood, especially the platelets, come into contact with the lining of the vessel and an aggregation of these forms a thrombus.

An individual undergoing surgery is at even greater risk, partly due to compression of the deep veins of the calf during the operation, and partly due to the changes which occur in the blood following surgery. The plasma becomes more viscous, its fibrinogen content increases, and the platelets cease to repel one another, tending to aggregate.

The thrombus may be firmly adherent to the blood vessel, the wall of which is inflamed, and acute pain in the calf and swelling of the limb are present. More dangerous is the thrombus which is not firmly adherent to the vessel wall, because symptoms and signs are difficult to detect and the thrombus may loosen from the wall of the vessel and be carried along with the flow of the blood. Between the leg veins and the heart the calibre of the vessels increases, but the vessels branch and decrease in diameter as the blood is distributed to the lungs. The thrombus may get lodged and occlude the blood vessels, causing a pulmonary infarction. If the infarction is sufficiently large, death may be instantaneous.

Prevention of deep vein thrombosis

The following factors help prevent deep vein thrombosis.

1. Leg exercises must be carried out frequently, at least hourly during the day. These consist of dorsi-flexion and plantar-flexion of the foot, against resistance. If the patient is unable to carry these out for himself, the ankle and knee joints should be taken passively through a full range of movement. The calf may also be massaged if the patient is unable to exercise. Any pain or tenderness experienced by the patient must be reported immediately.
2. Deep breathing exercises should be taught to the patient, and the nurse must encourage him to carry them out every hour during the day.
3. The patient should not lie in one position for any length of time.
4. Any device which could further slow the blood flow in the veins must be avoided. Pillows should never be placed under the knee or calf.
5. Antiembolic stockings may be used for patients at particular risk. These stockings may be applied as part of the preoperative preparation.

To prevent pulmonary emboli

The prevention of a pulmonary embolus depends upon the prevention of deep vein thrombosis. If the latter should occur, its early detection and treatment will help to prevent an embolus.

Signs of deep vein thrombosis are:

1. A slight rise in temperature.
2. A slowly increasing pulse rate, with our without a temperature rise.
3. Tenderness of the calf on local palpation.
4. Tenderness of the calf, if the foot is suddenly dorsi-flexed. This is called Homans' sign.

If deep vein thrombosis should occur, anticoagulants may be given, and if the physician considers that the danger of embolus formation is very great, then the vein may be occluded above the site of the thrombosis. The limb should be relieved of the weight of the bedclothes by the use of a cradle. A bandage or Tubigrip is usually applied to the limb.

12 Provision of rest and sleep: prevention of sensory deprivation or overload

In everyday life we alternate periods of activity with periods of rest. We also aim to get a good sleep every night and this pattern contributes to our sense of well-being. Obtaining rest and sleep is even more important for a person who is ill. Rest of the whole body and/or the affected part is the most common treatment prescribed by the physician, although it may be combined with other more specific forms of treatment. There is plenty of evidence to show that physical activity can disrupt healing tissue and that worry and anxiety delay healing.

The patient who remains at home when ill will at least sleep and rest in familiar surroundings. The patient will be well accustomed to the pattern of noise and activity within the neighbourhood, perhaps having lived there for many years. However, obtaining rest in a hospital ward is less easy than it sounds. In an open ward there is much activity, bustle and noise. To the staff a ward is their work place. Other patients may be noisy. Telephones ringing, the rattle of trolleys, conversation and possibly traffic noise are common features. In geriatric wards and long-stay wards the television or radio may be left on in the day room the whole time, regardless of whether anyone is interested in the programme. The survey of patients' attitudes carried out for the Royal Commission on the National Health Service (Gregory, 1978) found that 12% of adult patients spoken to were disturbed by noise during the daytime. Women were affected more than men. The disturbance was such as to prevent rest.

So far, discussion has centred on factors within the patient's environment (extrinsic factors) which impinge upon the patient preventing rest or causing distress. Factors within the individual (intrinsic factors) can also disturb the patients. Such factors as pain, discomfort, worries and anxieties can seriously disrupt a patient's rest. Nursing action must be designed to prevent such intrinsic factors, to identify them if they occur and to take nursing measures to alleviate them.

SENSORY DEPRIVATION AND OVERLOAD

Meaningful noise attracts attention and arouses the individual. Similarly, movement catches the eye and arouses attention. Both noise and movement constitute a form of sensory stimulation. Research has shown that the total level of sensory stimulation impinging upon an individual is important in relation to optimum psychological and physiological functioning. It does not matter too much which of the special senses is stimulated, through sight, sound, taste, smell or touch, but there is an optimum level of total stimulation for each individual. The optimum level may vary from time to time depending upon the activity in which a person is engaged, the general state of health, and age.

This means that there can be too little stimulation impinging on an individual, or there can be too much. A sparsity or impoverishment of stimulation is called sensory deprivation, whilst an excess is called sensory overload. Under normal circumstances, a healthy individual is able to seek out the optimum level of stimulation. If the environment is too noisy for rest or study, he moves to a quieter environment if possible. If the room is bare and unstimulating, he goes to where there is activity and movement or puts on the TV or plays tapes. A hospital patient cannot do this and so the nursing staff have to bear in mind the possibility of too much or too little sensory stimulation within the patient's environment.

From the point of view of patient care, a concept which is more important than sensory deprivation is that of perceptual deprivation. Sensory deprivation occurs when there is an absolute low level of stimulation from the environment. An example would be a silent, dark room where stimulation is limited to that engendered by the person himself through touch, movement and talking.

Perceptual deprivation can occur where there is noise and light but where the noise and the objects reflecting light are meaningless to the person. For example, a patient who had severe cataracts and who could not understand English might suffer from perceptual deprivation. So might an elderly patient placed in a day room with pop music playing all day, when the pop music just seems a meaningless jangle.

There are some patients who are especially at risk from sensory or perceptual deprivation; these include patients who are nursed in single rooms, those whose movement is curtailed by splints, and people who have to lie flat. Patients with hearing and visual defects, elderly patients and long-stay psychogeriatric patients are particularly at risk from a monotonous environment.

Nurses should also bear in mind the possibility of sensory overload in the case of some patients. This includes all patients on a busy, noisy, open ward. Patients being nursed in intensive care units are at risk from a simultaneous combination of sensory overload with perceptual deprivation. Intensive care units contain much strange-looking, noisy machinery which has little or no meaning for patients. Often the lights are left on day and night and sometimes there are no outside windows, giving no demarcation between night and day. The view the patient has may be very limited since the monitors, etc. restrict the ability to move. He may be unable to speak because of tracheostomy or endotracheal tube.

Under experimental conditions, normal, healthy volunteers may suffer hallucinations when subjected to perceptual or sensory deprivation. This show how important it is to prevent either of these conditions from occurring in patients.

SLEEP

Most of us have experienced at least one night of sleeplessness, and we know how tired we feel the following day. A good night's sleep helps us to feel rested and ready to face the day's activities and problems. Henderson (1964) said, 'Inability to rest and sleep is one of the causes as well as the accompaniment of disease'. Most of us accept that if sleep is important when we are well, it is even more important when we are ill.

Research has shown that sleep appears to be essential for normal physiological and psychological function. However, the amount of sleep a person needs is less clear cut. It seems to vary between individuals from 5 to 10 hours a night. It also seems to vary from time to time for any one individual, and certainly it varies at different points within one's life span. Babies appear to need a lot of sleep but the length of time they spend sleeping gradually becomes less until adult life. Beyond middle age the amount of sleep needed seems to get less again, but may increase in extreme old age. There also seems to be individual differences in the time at which a person needs to go to bed and get up in the morning. Some people seem to thrive on 'late nights' whilst others cope better with 'early nights' accompanied by early rising. Whilst some of the individual variation in sleep patterns seems to be inborn, there is little doubt that much variation is derived from habits and lifestyle.

The electroencephalogram (EEG) has been used to study sleep in human beings. This machine amplifies minute electrical currents picked up from the scalp and displays them on paper by means of an ink and pen recorder. Changes in the resultant wave pattern can be associated with the behavioural changes which occur. Volunteers sleep in a laboratory to allow such research to take place.

As an individual falls asleep, the pattern of deflections of the pen changes and the electrical activity appears to become synchronized. This is shown by larger and slower wave patterns on the paper, as the individual appears to be more and more deeply asleep. After a period of such 'slow wave sleep' (SWS), the wave pattern is broken, the synchrony is disturbed and the EEG begins to look rather as it does when a person is awake. However, to the watcher the individual is sleeping, but careful observation suggests that rapid eye movement (REM) is occurring under the lids. Special recording techniques have confirmed this. Movements of the eyeball are similar to those one makes whilst awake and watching something. If woken during this type of sleep, the person usually claims to have been dreaming. This type of sleep is called REM sleep. Periods of SWS get fewer and periods of REM sleep get greater as the night progresses. Research has shown that, if deprived of REM, the individual becomes irritable in the daytime. When allowed to sleep normally, a much greater length of time is spent in REM sleep than usual, as if making up for the deprivation.

Both types of sleep appear necessary for normal physical and mental health. By studying the hormonal and bio-chemical pattern associated with sleep, it is thought that SWS is associated with the cellular repair and growth of the body in general, whilst REM sleep is associated with the maintenance of the structure of the cells of the nervous system itself. REM sleep may also be associated with the laying down of memories. It can be seen from this brief account how important sleep is for recuperation.

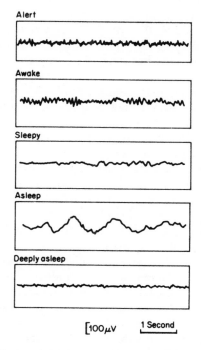

Alert

Awake

Sleepy

Asleep

Deeply asleep

$\lbrack 100\mu V$ 1 Second

Figure 12.1 Changes in the normal electroencephalogram.

The use of night sedation

People with insomnia are often prescribed night sedatives to help them to sleep. There are at least three problems associated with the use of night sedation. One is that with prolonged use the person develops increasing tolerance to the drugs, i.e. a larger dose is required to produce the same effect. The second problem also occurs as a result of prolonged use. It is that the individual may develop psychological and physiological dependence on the drug. Psychological dependence means that the person becomes anxious and stressful if the drug is not available and the anxiety and stress are immediately relieved on taking the drug. Physiological dependence means that the person's body structure has adapted to the presence of the drug and its withdrawal creates physiological disturbance. In the case of barbiturates, the withdrawal symptoms may take the form of epileptic fits.

Patients in hospital may be prescribed drugs to help them to sleep. It is important to realize that the two problems mentioned above are associated with the prolonged use of night sedatives and so they are unlikely to develop during a patient's stay in hospital. The third problem, however, arises even with the first dose of a night sedative. It is that most drugs interfere with the normal sleep pattern. The REM sleep in particular seems to be suppressed by night sedatives. Research shows that there is a so-called rebound effect when they are withdrawn. That is, for the first nights without the drug, REM sleep predominates and the individual complains of dreams and restlessness and even nightmares. The drug of choice as a night sedative is one of the benzodiazepine group. These are rapidly effective, they have little 'hangover' effect, and individuals rarely develop tolerance to them. They also interfere little with normal sleep waves.

Factors interfering with sleep

In caring for patients, a nurse will be concerned to provide conditions which are conducive to sleep. Both intrinsic and extrinsic factors may interfere with sleep.

Extrinsic factors

Researchers carrying out the patient attitude survey for the Royal Commission on the National Health Service (1978) asked their sample about sleeping in hospital. Twenty-seven per cent said they had been generally disturbed during the night, and for half of these the disturbance made it difficult to get even a 'fair' night's sleep. The greater the number of beds in the ward, the higher the proportion of patients who said they had been disturbed. Reasons for the disturbance included the noise made by other patients and emergency admissions. However, some patients complained of the noise made by staff and the lights which were left on for the convenience of the staff. There were even complaints from a few patients that they had been woken up by nurses checking to see if they were asleep! One in eight of patients found the hospital bed uncomfortable and complained particularly of the plastic draw sheet which made them feel hot. Rough, stiff sheets also caused discomfort.

The survey also confirmed that patients generally were woken very early in the morning. Over 40% of patients were woken by 6 a.m. It was worse for maternity patients, 36% of whom were woken between 5 a.m. and 5.30 a.m., and 32% between 5.30 and 6 a.m. Not surprisingly, nearly half the patients questioned complained of being woken too early. More women than men felt they were woken too early.

Apart from the finding of this survey, most of us develop

habits at bed time which help us to get to sleep. It is unlikely that sleep routines can be maintained in hospital. After all, many people take alcohol in the evening, which undoubtedly helps them to sleep! Familiar surroundings help sleep and the very unfamiliarity of the hospital ward can interfere with sleep. Unusual times of settling for the night also require a good deal of adjustment on the patient's part. Patients being cared for in their own homes can maintain their usual time of settling to sleep. However, intrinsic factors may interfere with their sleep patterns.

Intrinsic factors

Factors within the patient likely to interfere with sleep include those likely to interfere with rest in the daytime, such as pain, discomfort, worries, anxieties and fears. In addition, feeling hungry or wanting to pass urine may interfere with sleep. Patients who have to be nursed in a special position may find this interferes with sleep. Usually, we all have a favourite position in which to sleep and a different position makes sleep more difficult.

Assessment

Ideally, assessment includes a note of the environment for care and the extent to which environmental factors are likely to interfere with rest or sleep. It is equally important to identify those patients particularly at risk from sensory deprivation or overload. Assessment is carried out to provide information so that the environment can be matched as well as possible with the patient's needs. Obviously it may be difficult to modify the hospital ward environment except in small ways, but it is possible to choose carefully the position in the ward in which a patient's bed is placed. For patients in their own home, the community nurse can advise about the provision of modifications to the sleeping environment which would aid sleep. During assessment, consideration should be given to the following points.

1. Is the patient used to a noisy, bustling environment (e.g. a factory) or is he normally in a very quiet rural environment?
2. Is the patient's sensory input restricted in any way through defects of vision, hearing, smell, taste, touch or through restriction of movement?
3. How much can the patient see from the bed position?
4. Is it likely that the patient can hear noise from machinery without being able to see or understand the noise?
5. How ill does the patient feel, since the worse he feels the more his need for rest and quiet?
6. Is rest a part of the patient's prescribed treatment?
7. If the patient is sleeping in the day, can the treatment or meal wait until he wakes up?
8. Can several procedures be carried out consecutively so that there is a long period of peace without disturbance for nursing care?
9. Is there a patient in the ward who is particularly noisy? Is it possible to move the noisy patient to a position where disturbance to other patients will be less, or to use any other nursing measure to quieten the patient?

Assessment at night

1. Does the patient normally take night sedation at home? If so, what is taken?
2. Is the patient normally used to traffic noise at night or is the bedroom very quiet?
3. Is the patient used to sleeping away from home in hotels or boarding houses?

4. At what time does the patient normally go to bed and wake up?
5. What position does the patient normally assume for sleeping?
6. Does nursing have to be in one special position?
7. Does the patient really need a plastic draw sheet or can it be removed for the night?
8. Does he need a hot drink?
9. Does he need to use the toilet?
10. Is he worried or anxious about anything?
11. Does he need to talk to someone?
12. Does he have any pain or discomfort?
13. Is the ward temperature too hot or too cold and does the patient have the right number of bedclothes on his bed?
14. What is the best time to administer a sleeping pill if one has been prescribed?
15. If the patient had difficulty in falling asleep, can morning treatments and observations be left until he wakes naturally?

Care of the patient during the daytime

The aim of care is: (1) to help the patient to obtain the rest needed, whilst preventing the complications of immobility; and (2) to help the patient to obtain the optimum level of stimulation in the light of the illness and stage of recovery.

A general measure is to remind all staff to be as quiet as possible at all times, to ensure the maintenance of equipment so it runs smoothly and quietly, and to plan each patient's nursing care individually to prevent unnecessary disturbance. Arranging pillows comfortably and giving analgesia to relieve pain and discomfort are important aspects of nursing care. All procedures should be carefully explained to each patient. Staff should be sensitive to cues that the patient is worried or anxious and arrangements should be made for a sympathetic member of staff to sit and encourage the patient to talk. Visiting from relatives should be encouraged.

Patients who are at risk from monotony in hospital can be encouraged to go to the day room where there is a TV and other patients to talk to. If a group of patients is together in the day room, staff could encourage group discussions or carry out some health education. Nursing staff or voluntary workers can be encouraged to sit and talk to patients, and relatives encouraged to visit as frequently as possible. Young orthopaedic patients may suffer particularly from monotony. In children's wards nurses are encouraged to play with patients, but in adult wards orthopaedic patients could perhaps be encouraged to have a personal radiocassette player with earphones of the 'Walkman' type. Books, magazines or packs of cards may also be useful to entertain patients. Some patients may like to have facilities to do some study in hospital.

Care at night

The aim of care is to allow each patient to have a good night's sleep, preferably without the intervention of sedative drugs. If at all possible, the ward atmosphere should be quiet, calm and peaceful in the hour leading to lights out. During this time milky drinks are usually dispensed, toilet facilities offered and patients' beds made comfortable. When lights are put out, any left on for the staff's convenience must be kept to a minimum and shaded. Staff should be as quiet as possible in their movements and avoid knocking things or banging doors. Quiet shoes should be worn. Any squeaking doors should be reported so that the hinges can be oiled.

If a patient is having difficulty in sleeping, his comfort should be attended to. If a patient appears anxious or upset, he should be encouraged to talk quietly without disturbing other patients. A mobile patient could be taken to the kitchen or day room if there is a need to talk. Any pain should be relieved by the administration of prescribed drugs. Night sedation should be given if prescribed and if the patient wants it. Any patient who had difficulty in getting off to sleep should be allowed to sleep on undisturbed in the morning if at all possible.

The nurse's skill will be reflected in a report that the patient slept well.

13 Care of the patient with problems of respiration

One of the most basic requirements for life to continue is to be able to breathe. By breathing, we maintain both the oxygen and the carbon dioxide levels in the blood within acceptable limits. Oxygen is used in each cell of the body in combination with nutrients to produce energy. Energy is needed by every cell for the maintenance of the integrity of its own structure, for cell division, and in carrying out the special function of the cell. Examples of the energy use in special functions include muscle cells which use energy in contraction, nerve cells which use energy in maintaining the nerve potential which is vital for the nerve impulse, and endocrine cells which use energy in the production of hormones.

Carbon dioxide is produced by cells as a by-product of the oxidation of nutrients. Although if it accumulates within a cell or in the immediate environment of the cell it depresses its activity, it is important to note that the presence of carbon dioxide in the blood plays an important role in the maintenance of respiration and in the maintenance of an optimum acid—base balance (pH).

ASSESSMENT OF RESPIRATORY FUNCTION

Assessment of respiratory function may have to be carried out instantaneously as life-saving action is initiated to maintain the oxygen level of the blood. The cessation of respirations must be immediately identified and artificial respiration carried out (unless otherwise instructed). Obstruction of the respiratory tract is also an emergency and it must be relieved straight away or the patient will die. Noisy respirations are the indicator of some greater or lesser degree of obstruction. The obstruction must be identified and dealt with, but in the meantime oxygen can be given if the obstruction is partial. Possible causes of respiratory obstruction include the tongue, vomit, secretions, displaced dentures in unconscious patients, laryngeal spasm or a foreign body. In the case of the last two causes, an emergency tracheostomy may well be needed.

Less dramatic circumstances in which respiratory assessment may be carried out allow attention to be directed to the following points.

1. Does the patient have any pain in the chest, if so is it continuous; on inspiration; or on expiration?
2. Note if respiratory movement is equal on both sides of the chest and if breathing is mainly diaphragmatic, intercostal or both. Are the respiratory movements laboured in any way and are the accessory muscles of respiration brought into use?
3. Can the patient breathe easily whilst lying flat or does he have to sit up? Check the rate of respirations.
4. Note the patient's colour. Does he look pink and healthy or does the skin look grey? Is there any cyanosis and if so is it confined to the periphery? Is it central? Or both? Note any clubbing of the fingers.
5. The patient should be asked if there is any coughing. If so, when does it occur? Is it dry, or does he expectorate freely? Any sputum should be observed for colour, consistency and quantity.
6. Does the patient get asthmatic attacks? If so, under

what circumstances? What is taken for attacks? How severe are they?

7. Does the patient appear to have sinusitis, a head cold, or a sore throat? Is the voice at all husky and if so has it always been like that?

8. The body temperature should be recorded.

CARE OF THE PATIENT WITH RESPIRATORY PROBLEMS

One of the most important measures of nursing care to help a patient with a respiratory problem is to place him in the correct position. A position in which he sits up well, amply supported by pillows, helps good expansion of the chest on inspiration. The semi-prone or head-down position helps the drainage of secretions from the chest. Lying on the left side helps expansion of the right lung and vice versa.

An asthmatic patient may well appreciate having the bed placed near a window which will open.

Deep breathing exercises will be taught to patients who are particularly at risk for the development of chest infection.

A patient with a head cold or a dry cough may find steam inhalations helpful in soothing inflamed membranes. Inhalations may be given routinely to some patients post-operatively to help to moisten particulate matter in the respiratory passages so that it can be coughed up.

Steam inhalation

When a patient has an upper respiratory tract infection such as laryngitis, pharyngitis or a head cold, a steam inhalation may relieve symptoms. The treatment can be given by means of a Nelson's inhaler. It should be half filled with boiling water to which a prescribed quantity of Friar's Balsam or menthol can be added. A flannel hot water bottle cover should be wrapped around the inhaler, and the latter should be placed in a bowl. The whole apparatus should be on a firm surface, such as a table, for the patient's use. There must be no danger that it might tip, and if the patient cannot cooperate, the inhaler must not be left in the vicinity, unsupervised by staff.

A gauze swab should be fixed in position with adhesive tape round the glass mouthpiece, and the patient is instructed to put the lips to the mouthpiece and breathe in through the mouth and out through the nose. The treatment is continued until the water cools. Mouthpieces must be sterilized between use.

A satisfactory substitute for a Nelson's inhaler can be made by using a litre jug. A towel is placed round the rim and the patient is instructed to lean forward and breathe the steam.

OXYGEN

Oxygen benefits the patient whose respiratory capacity is diminished, as is the case following chest injuries or operations on the lung, in pneumonia, acute pulmonary oedema, cardiac failure and many other conditions.

Oxygen cylinders and fittings

For purposes of identification, oxygen and other medical gas cylinders are painted in distinctive colours and the name and/or symbol of the gas is stencilled on the cylinder. Oxygen cylinders are painted black with a white valve end.

Oxygen is compressed into cylinders of different sizes at 13 332 kPa. This pressure must be reduced prior to administration to a patient. Wherever possible an automatic oxygen regulator should be employed for this purpose, but when not available a fine adjustment valve may be used with care. A litre gauge or flowmeter is necessary in order that the prescribed rate of flow may be maintained. These gauges may be of the dial or the bobbin type. In the latter a bobbin inside a graduated glass tube rises as the oxygen passes through and the height of the bobbin against the scale shows the amount of oxygen being delivered. The flowmeter is usually incorporated in the cylinder fitting with the pressure gauge and regulator.

Before attaching the regulator to the cylinder, the cylinder valve should be opened slightly, so that any grit or dust that may have accumulated may be blown out. The regulator is then fitted into the head of the cylinder by inserting the threaded end into the valve opening and tightening it by means of the winged nut. The litre gauge should be turned off and the cylinder opened slowly until the cylinder contents gauge shows 'full', the cylinder is then opened completely by giving the key one more turn. The cylinder is then ready for use.

In many wards the oxygen supply may be delivered by a pipeline to each bed, but every ward should possess at least one oxygen outfit ready for immediate use. The cylinder, in a wheeled stand with the fittings, and the apparatus for delivering the oxygen to the patient, should be regarded as emergency apparatus which must always be kept in working order. An empty cylinder should be clearly marked 'EMPTY' when removed from the stand and should be replaced at once by a full cylinder.

Fire precautions

Although oxygen itself does not burn, any material which burns in atmospheric air will burn much more easily if the concentration of oxygen in the air is increased. Therefore, certain precautions should be strictly observed.

Patients and visitors should be warned against smoking or lighting matches in the vicinity. No electrical bells, lights or heating pads should be allowed inside an oxygen tent and children should not be given mechanical toys. The patient must not be rubbed with oil or spirit whilst the tent is being operated; should such procedure be necessary, the oxygen flow must be discontinued during the time that the treatment is being carried out.

Oil or grease of any description must not be used on the oxygen cylinder or fittings. Oil and grease are inflammable. They may also dry out causing a blockage in the apparatus. The nozzle of the cylinder must be cleaned before attaching the regulator.

Administration of oxygen

Oxygen may be given by means of a mask, an oxygen tent or through nasal tubes or fine catheters. Whenever a patient is having oxygen therapy he must be under continuous observation. The apparatus must be frequently and carefully checked; should the supply of oxygen run out, the patient may be unable to obtain sufficient air. In certain cases, for example in patients suffering from chronic bronchitis and emphysema who develop pneumonia, carbon dioxide may build up in the blood when the anoxia, which has been the respiratory stimulus in these patients, has been relieved. This can lead to carbon dioxide narcosis, the symptoms of which are a full bounding pulse, muscular twitchings, mental confusion and eventually coma. For this reason intermittent rather than continuous oxygen is usually ordered for bronchitic subjects, or oxygen may be administered by Venti mask (see below).

Masks

Disposable polythene mask. A polythene mask is light in weight and as it is inexpensive it can be destroyed after use and so presents no problems of sterilization. When the mask is connected to the oxygen supply, the flow of oxygen inflates a cuff round the edge of the mask, which then fits closely and comfortably. Should the oxygen supply accidentally run out, the cuff will deflate, thus calling attention to the failure; in the meantime the patient can continue to breathe atmospheric air.

The Ventimask. (Figure 13.1). The Ventimask is designed to give accurate control of the oxygen concentration so that it does not rise high enough to cause respiratory depression, but is sufficient to relieve anoxia. The range of controlled concentration is 24–35%. The disposable face piece is edged with foam rubber so that it fits closely and comfortably round the patient's nose.

Tracheostomy mask. (Figure 13.2). If a patient has had a tracheostomy performed, it is obvious that he cannot benefit from oxygen given through a face mask. The

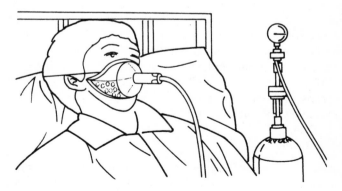

Figure 13.1 A Ventimask

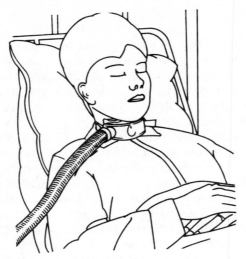

Figure 13.2 A tracheostomy mask.

tracheostomy mask shown in the illustration is made of perspex and fits over the tracheostomy opening; an opening with a peardrop cover in the front of the mask, over the tube, allows suction to be carried out with the mask in position. There are perforations at the side of the mask; these allow excess carbon dioxide to be removed and enable the patient to breathe atmospheric air, should the oxygen supply fail.

If a mask is not available, oxygen can be given by means of a catheter passed through the opening of the tracheostomy tube.

Nasal tubes

Administration of oxygen by nasal tube is used if a tent is not available or a face mask is not suitable, as, for example, where there are facial injuries. It is much less efficient than either the tent or the mask as it is wasteful of oxygen and the patient cannot as a rule tolerate a rate of flow greater than 4 litres/minute. Disposable nasal tubes are used.

When giving oxygen by nasal tube it is necessary to moisten the oxygen by passing it through a humidifier before it reaches the patient, as dry oxygen is irritating to the nasal passages.

Before the tubes are inserted the nostrils should be cleaned with warm sodium bicarbonate lotion and wool swabs. A cocaine spray or cocaine ointment may be used in order to make the treatment less uncomfortable for the patient. The two nasal tubes should be passed about 5 cm along the floor of the nostrils. The tubes should be removed and cleaned if left in for more than 24 hours.

TRACHEOSTOMY

A tracheostomy is an artificial opening into the trachea, which is kept patent by the insertion of a metal or Portex tube (Figure 13.3). It may have been created as an emerg-

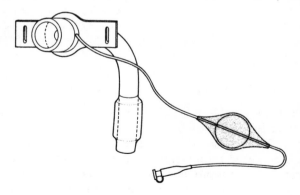

Figure 13.3 Cuffed tracheostomy tube.

ency operation or it may have been planned and carried out in more ideal conditions with the patient having had time to adjust to the idea of the operation.

Reasons for tracheostomy

1. In respiratory obstruction if the obstruction is above the tracheostomy site.
2. If there is paralysis of the vocal cords.
3. To aid suction of secretions from the respiratory tract, in respiratory tract infection.
4. To reduce the respiratory dead space so that more efficient exchange of respiratory gases can occur.
5. To ensure maximum efficiency of the system if the patient is being artificially respired with a positive pressure respirator.

Types of tracheostomy tube

Silver tube

A silver tube has both an outer tube, and an inner tube. The latter can be removed for cleaning at frequent intervals. The outer tube should be removed every 7 days by a member of the medical staff, and replaced by a new, sterile set.

Portex inflatable tube

A Portex inflatable tube is disposable and does not have an inner tube. It does have an inflatable cuff around the lumen. The cuff should not be inflated unless an airtight seal is required to prevent aspiration of saliva and other secretions or to provide intermittent positive pressure ventilation. In this case, only the minimum pressure for an airtight fit should be supplied. The pressure should be checked and adjusted by an anaesthetist once a day (Bevan, 1975). A Portex tube which fits into the trachea but has no inflatable cuff may also be used occasionally.

Equipment which should be kept at the bedside

- Suction machine or piped suction; the tubing should be fitted with a polythene 'Y' connection
- Oxygen cylinder or piped oxygen
- A pair of sterile dressing forceps
- Suction catheters of the correct size
- A bowl of sterile sodium bicarbonate solution
- Disposable gloves
- Sterile tracheal dilator forceps
- Sterile tracheostomy set of appropriate type and an introducer
- Syringe and adaptor if a cuffed tracheostomy tube is in use
- For a conscious patient, a bell and writing materials

Care of the airway

It is vital that the patient's airway should be kept clear. Signs that the airway is becoming blocked are as follows.

1. In the early stages, the respirations become noisy. This is the stage at which the situation should be detected and dealt with.
2. The patient may become cyanosed in colour.
3. If the hand is placed directly in front of the tube, no air can be felt on expiration.

Action to be taken

For partial blockage, suction may be employed to clear the airway. If there is an inner tube present, it should be removed for cleaning, and suction should be carried out through the outer tube. If neither of these measures works, then the patient should be positioned with the head retracted and the neck extended, and the outer tube should be removed. Tracheal dilators should be inserted to maintain the opening and suction should be carried out, through the neck incision. Medical help will be required to insert another tube. Oxygen can be given, and artificial respiration may be necessary. The obstruction must be relieved as rapidly as possible.

Routine maintenance of the airway

Since it will be extremely difficult for the patient to cough, suction should be carried out at intervals sufficiently frequent to prevent distress of the patient.

Suction of a patient with a tracheostomy

To carry out suction, the following steps should be taken.

1. Have the patient lying on the back with the head retracted and the neck extended. Full explanation should be given.
2. Choose an appropriate suction catheter which is only half the diameter of the tracheostomy tube. It should have an opening in the end, across the diameter of the catheter.
3. Use disposable gloves.
4. Open the pack containing the catheter and connect the end of the 'Y' connection of the suction apparatus.
5. Withdraw the catheter from the packet, using the left hand to hold it at the connection and a pair of sterile forceps in the right hand to grip the catheter near the other end.
6. Pass the catheter into the trachea, using the forceps.
7. Switch on the suction and occlude the open arm of the 'Y' connection.

8. If suction does not proceed smoothly, switch off the machine, withdraw the catheter, and use a fresh catheter, discarding the used one. Repeat from step (2). Continue the procedure until the patient's airway is clear.

9. Disconnect the catheter and dispose of it, together with the gloves. Make the patient comfortable. Throughout the procedure observation should be made of the patient's colour. Oxygen should be given if he becomes at all distressed.

Frequent turning and chest physiotherapy will help to loosen secretions. At least once a day 'artificial coughing' or 'bag-squeezing' should be carried out. This requires an anaesthetist, nurse and physiotherapist. The tracheostomy is connected via a catheter mount, expiratory valve and reservoir bag to a source of oxygen. The anaesthetist hyperventilates the patient for three to four 'breaths' with the expiratory valve almost closed. Chest movements are followed by the physiotherapist who has placed her hands on the patient's chest. After a deep inspiration the anaesthetist suddenly releases pressure on the reservoir bag and if this is combined with firm compression and vibration of the chest by the physiotherapist, it results in an explosive expiration. The debris can then be sucked from the trachea by the nurse using an aseptic technique. The procedure should be repeated for each area of the chest, accompanied by changes in the position of the patient (Bevan, 1975).

Humidification of inspired air

Humidification of inspired air is necessary to prevent the development of chest infection as the warm moist mucous membrane of the upper respiratory tract is no longer available to perform this function. Humidification may be carried out by means of a humidifier which warms as well as moistens the inspired air. The air as it reaches the patient should be moist and warm. The temperature should be 30–35°C (86–95°F). Moist gauze placed over the tracheostomy is an inefficient method of humidifying the inspired air. An alternative method is by a slow saline drip into the tracheostomy to provide 15–20 ml/h. Careful observation is required to ensure that this rate is not exceeded.

A thermal humidifying filter (Trach-Vent) (Figure 13.4)

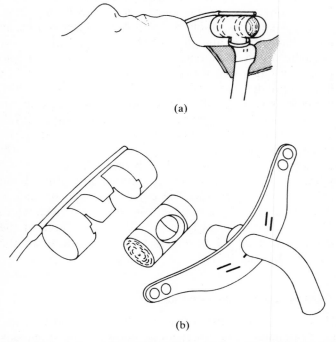

(a)

(b)

Figure 13.4 A thermal humidifying filter: (a) in position; (b) exploded view.

made by Portex connects directly to the 15-mm termination of the tracheostomy tube and maintains 85% relative humidity in the trachea at 37°C. The filter needs to be replaced every 24 hours, or as needed, to prevent accumulation of secretions.

An oxygen attachment may be used and clips directly over the Trach-Vent and supplies oxygen-enriched air which is warmed and humidified as it passes through the Trach-Vent.

POSITIVE PRESSURE RESPIRATORS

If artificial aid to breathing is required over a long period, some form of respirator is used, and most commonly this is a positive pressure respirator. With this respirator, gas is forced into the lungs under pressure at regular intervals, through a mask, an endotracheal tube, or a tracheostomy tube. Expiration either occurs passively, or by negative pressure. Types of respirator in common use include the Engstrom, Cape Wain, Bennet and Brompton-Manley. A nurse asked to work on a ward where one of these respirators is available for emergency use should ensure that she understands how it works at the beginning of the ward experience.

Observations to make on taking over the care of a patient being artificially respired include the following:

1. Observe the patient's colour and chest movement. The chest should inflate equally on either side.
2. Test all tubing for air leaks, and make sure that it is not kinked.
3. Check that you know how to operate the machine by hand in an emergency, and that you know how to give artificial respiration manually, if necessary. (An Ambu bag or similar apparatus should be available.)

4. Check that you are fully conversant with all the controls of the machine, and that the readings conform to those ordered by the doctor. Readings which must be checked carefully include the maximum and minimum pressure to be exerted by the machine, the respiratory rate required, tidal volume required, and possibly the expired minute volume.

5. If oxygen is being used, ensure that a supply is available and check the rate of flow.

6. If humidification of the air or oxygen is needed, check the temperature and that the humidifier is filled.

All these observations should be repeated at prescribed intervals.

In addition, the following points should be kept in mind:

1. If the patient should make respiratory movements which are out of phase with the machine, the doctor must be informed.

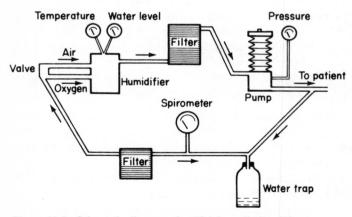

Figure 13.5 Schematic diagram of artificial ventilation (*Nursing Times*).

2. Great care must be taken not to disconnect the tubing when carrying out nursing care. After suction, make sure that the ventilator is properly reconnected (Figure 13.5).
3. If the pressure readings change, the cause should be traced and dealt with.

A rise in pressure may be due to obstruction to the flow of gas. This may be kinked tubing, an obstructed airway requiring suction, or, if the humidifier is in use, water may accumulate in the tubing. A fall in pressure is usually due to loss of gas from the system, so the tubing must be checked for leaks. The doctor should be notified if the situation cannot be corrected.

WATER-SEAL DRAINS

If the visceral and parietal pleural membranes are separated from each other by a collection of fluid or air, a drain may be inserted to drain these off by gravity and allow re-expansion of the lung. The free end of the drain must be sealed under water placed in a container well below the level of the patient, otherwise air would be sucked into the pleural cavity at each inspiration. Provided the tubing is patent and the lung has not fully re-expanded, the level of the water in the tubing (as it passes down into the bottle) rises, as the patient breathes in, and falls again as he breathes out.

This 'swinging' of the water level is, therefore, a good guide as to whether the tubing is patent and the reason should be investigated if the rise and fall cannot be seen. The amount of fluid draining in should be measured as necessary. A known and accurately measured quantity of fluid is placed in a fresh, sterile, bottle (Figure 13.6). To change the bottle, the tubing must first be clamped with

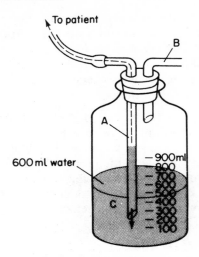

Figure 13.6 A drainage bottle with underwater seal. A, Tube connected to drainage tubing; B, air inlet tube; C, water seal. The air inlet tube (B) may be connected to another water seal bottle or suction apparatus. The principles of nursing management remain the same.

two pairs of Spencer Wells forceps placed near to the insertion of the tubing, to prevent air getting into the pleural cavity. Careful technique is essential to prevent microorganisms from getting into the apparatus. At no time must the water-seal bottle be lifted higher than, or even to a level with, the patient. This is because gravity would cause the fluid from the water-seal bottle to pass down the tubing to the patient's pleural cavity, with fatal consequences. The drainage tube is removed by the medical staff when the lung is fully re-expanded.

14 Maintenance of optimum body temperature

In health, and in all except the very young and the very old, the core body temperature stays within very narrow limits, in spite of wide variations in environmental temperature. *Core temperature* refers to the temperature within the skull, the heart, the thorax and the abdominal organs. *Peripheral temperature* refers to the body surface and the limbs. Peripheral temperature does vary according to the environmental temperature.

Maintenance of core temperature within a narrow range is dependent upon efficient functioning of the structures within the body which are associated with temperature homeostasis. However, even in the healthy young adult extremely adverse environmental temperature can lead to changes in core body temperature. It is the thermo-regulatory centre within the hypothalamus which exerts control upon core body temperature. This centre behaves as if it has a 'set point' temperature to guide thermo-regulation. If the actual core temperature is lower than this, then mechanisms come into play which conserve and/or produce body heat. On the other hand, if the actual core temperature is higher than the set point, then those mechanisms which help in the loss of body heat come into action.

Clearly, in order to exert control the hypothalamus must receive information relating to the current body temperature. This comes from at least two sources. One is from cells within the hypothalamus itself which monitor the temperature of the blood flowing through the hypothalamus. (There may be similar monitoring in other parts of the central nervous system.) The other information source is from sensory fibres responding to temperature within the skin. It is believed that the central receptors respond to heat and help in the defence against temperature rise, whilst the peripheral skin receptors monitor cold, in particular. An interaction between the central and peripheral information then helps to guard against temperature fall. The hypothalamus exerts control through biochemical and physiological responses. In man, behavioural responses are also important in temperature homeostasis.

RESPONSES WHICH PROTECT AGAINST A FALL IN CORE BODY TEMPERATURE

Behavioural

These include:

1. Wearing warm clothing
2. Taking exercise
3. Huddling near to a source of heat

in cold conditions

4. In addition we tend to eat more warm and high calorie foods, although the effect of this action is fairly short-lived.

Physiological

1. Skin vasoconstriction prevents heat loss from radiation, conduction and evaporation.
2. Shivering may occur and increases heat production from muscular activity.

3. A counter-current heat exchange mechanism operates in the limbs, particularly the legs. A network of veins around the arteries allows heat to pass from the arteries into venous blood returning to the heart, thus conserving core temperature.

Biochemical

1. Increased secretion of adrenaline and noradrenaline act to increase the metabolic rate and thus heat production within the body. This mechanism may help to protect the body against cold but it tends to be short lived.
2. Thyroxine, secreted by the thyroid gland in response to thyroid stimulating hormone from the hypothalamus, also increases the metabolic rate, but this is not believed to be of practical importance in man in relation to environmental temperature.
3. Brown fat occurs around the back of the neck and kidneys in infants. As its name implies it appears darker than the normal fat of adults. Brown fat cells contain more mitochondria and the fat globules are more easily and rapidly mobilized than white fat, releasing heat more readily. It is questionable whether brown fat is retained into adult life but it provides a good source of heat in infants.

RESPONSES WHICH PROTECT AGAINST A RISE IN CORE BODY TEMPERATURE

Behavioural

Behavioural responses protecting against a rise in core body temperature during hot environmental conditions include:

1. Choosing suitable lightweight, absorbent clothing.
2. Tending to avoid heavy physical activity and to adopt a 'spread out' posture when inactive; this exposes the maximum amount of body surface to the air.
3. Reducing food intake; food and drink which is taken tends to be cold.

Physiological

1. The main physiological response allowing increased heat loss from the body is dilatation of skin blood vessels. When this dilatation occurs, warm blood flows near the body surface allowing heat to be lost by convection, conduction and radiation. Whilst conduction is of minor importance, about 70% of body heat is lost through these three physical procedures. Skin vasodilatation also allows evaporation of sweat to occur and sweating is greater under such conditions. Heat from the skin is the energy source for evaporation of sweat. However evaporation varies with the humidity of the air; the higher the humidity, the smaller the amount of evaporated sweat which can be accepted.
2. In addition to these processes of heat loss, some heat is lost in urine, faeces and expired air.

IMPLICATIONS OF THERMOREGULATORY MECHANISMS FOR THE MAINTENANCE OF HEALTH

In the absence of disease, there are two main potential problems to guard against in relation to temperature homeostasis. These are heat stroke and hypothermia. In addition, heat exhaustion, frost-bite and the dangers of overexposure to natural or artificial sunlight will be mentioned.

Hypothermia

Two groups of people who are particularly vulnerable to hypothermia are infants and the elderly. Central mechanisms guarding the core temperature are less efficient at the extremes of age. To consider infants first: the main danger is from cold bedrooms, especially if the infant throws bed-covers off. The British climate in particular can vary very rapidly overnight from being mild to becoming very cold. Clearly, infants also need to be well protected from cold and damp when out of doors. Their clothing needs to be chosen with care. Poor families may be tempted to economize both on heating and clothing.

Elderly people on low incomes may also be tempted to use heating very sparingly. They may also be very inactive due to disability. Old people who fall in the home and fail to attract attention can develop hypothermia quite rapidly.

People whose age falls between the two extremes may be in danger of hypothermia under adverse environmental conditions. Clearly, being stranded out of doors in snow is an example, but so is being outside in wet clothes when conditions are both cold and windy. Similarly, being plunged into cold water out of doors is hazardous. Homeless people, sleeping rough, are also potentially vulnerable to hypothermia.

Frost-bite

Frost-bite can occur when an individual is exposed to low environmental temperatures. It affects peripheral areas in particular, e.g. toes, fingers, lips, nose and ears. Prevention involves the use of warm socks, shoes, gloves, and a scarf to cover the vulnerable areas of the face.

Heat stroke

Prior to the consideration of heat stroke it is useful to draw attention to the importance of the temperature of the tissues within the skull. Hypothalamic cells controlling body temperature are vulnerable to a high temperature in the blood supply to the hypothalamus and their thermo-regulatory function can be affected. In practice, a counter-current system operates in relation to the head, helping to maintain a constant temperature within the skull. The jugular veins drawing blood from the head lie adjacent to the carotid arteries within the neck. The latter vessels carry blood to the brain. The anatomical arrangement facilitates heat exchange between the two vessels.

Direct heat radiating to the skull, neck or spinal column can increase the local temperature of nervous tissue and/ or its blood supply. This leads to the condition of heat stroke. Heat stroke can also occur in high environmental temperatures when the body cannot lose heat rapidly enough; for example, in high humidity. As the body temperature rises, so does the metabolic rate and therefore extra heat from endogenous sources exacerbates matters. It is important, therefore, to avoid direct heat to the neck and head, such as direct sunlight streaming down. In hot environments the use of a fan may supplement open doors, windows, etc. when air conditioning is not available.

Heat exhaustion

Heat exhaustion can be distinguished from heat stroke. It is due to excessive sweating in high environmental temperature with a consequent loss of liquid and electrolyte unless replacement drinks are taken.

Exposure of skin to natural or artificial sunlight

Whilst not strictly relevant to our discussion of temperature homeostasis, it is convenient to mention here the dangers of excessive exposure to natural or artificial sun-rays (ultra-violet light) to fair-skinned people without gradual ac-climatization. The danger is two-fold: short-term and long-term. In the short term, exposure can lead to red, dry, blistering and peeling skin which can be painful. This effect usually passes and the skin heals satisfactorily. In the long term, the probability of developing melanoma (a malignant condition of the skin) increases with excessive exposure to ultraviolet light. Prevention of the condition is the avoidance of exposure of the skin to the ultraviolet rays. This, of course, is difficult in a sunny climate and many people in less sunny climates see it as desirable to go to the sun for a holiday and to get a tan as quickly as possible. Advice here is to expose the skin to the sun for only short periods, using a protective cream which filters out ultraviolet rays. In the long term, a strategy of health education to bring about attitude change is the current policy.

Significance of choice of clothing

As mentioned above, clothing plays an important part in man's behavioural control of body temperature. Like some other forms of behaviour which have evolved in relation to survival, clothing has acquired a cultural signifi-cance far beyond its instrumental purpose. Individuals vary in relation to the significance which they attribute both to their own and other's clothing. However, among the cultural and psychological functions performed by clothing are included modesty, sexual display, expression of personality, identification with a specific social or professional group, dignity and sexual identification. Clothing becomes a part of the total person and may influence to a large extent our first impressions of an individual.

All these possible functions which clothing may perform should be borne in mind in relation to patient care. Normally, on admission to hospital, during one of the first interactions with nursing staff, a patient is asked to remove his or her day clothes and change into night clothes. This immediately differentiates patients from staff or visitors and may place the patient psychologically at a disadvantage in relation to persons who are fully clothed.

Another circumstance in which nurses need to bear in mind the importance of clothing is in long-stay accommodation or wards. Frequently, people who are incontinent of urine are asked to wear institutionally-owned clothing rather than their own, due to the difficulty of providing individual laundry services. This practice is degrading and potentially dehumanizing. Every effort should be made to enable patients to wear their own clothing.

The remainder of this chapter will be devoted to a more specific outline of nursing intervention in the care of patients with problems related to temperature regulation.

THE CARE OF PATIENTS WITH PYREXIA

An increase in body temperature occurs when there is an initial increase in heat production and a decrease in loss of heat from the body.

Factors which increase heat production are:

1. Increased secretion of adrenaline.
2. Increased secretion of thyroxine.
3. Increased muscular activity, as in rigor.

Factors which decrease heat loss are:

1. Vasoconstriction of peripheral blood vessels.
2. Diminished sweating.

The following disease processes may be associated with pyrexia.

1. Infection and inflammation due to microorganisms.
2. Tissue infarction.
3. Haemorrhage.
4. Collagen disease.
5. Malignant disease.
6. Reaction to foreign protein.
7. Lesions of the brain stem and hypothalamus.

In all of these conditions, with the exception of the last named, cells in the hypothalamic thermoregulatory centre are depressed by circulating 'pyrogens', either directly or via prostaglandins, and act as if they are 'reset' to control the temperature at a higher level than normal.

As well as the conditions listed above, an increase in the amount of circulating thyroid hormones will cause a rise in body temperature by a direct effect on metabolism.

The effects of pyrexia upon the body

1. The basal metabolic rate is increased by 7% for each half degree celsius (one degree Fahrenheit, approximately) rise of temperature above the normal.
2. There is an increase in the pulmonary ventilation rate and the cardiac output.
3. Since the basal metabolic rate is increased, there may be excessive protein breakdown, a tendency to ketosis and negative nitrogen balance, unless the energy intake is adequate to counteract this. If protein breakdown

does occur, body wasting may result from prolonged pyrexia.
4. An increase in sweating may occur after the initial rise of temperature and this may be sufficient to cause sodium and fluid depletion.

Hyperpyrexia is a particularly dangerous condition, since above a body temperature of 41°C (106°F), the temperature-controlling centre itself may fail, and death may ensue if the high temperature is prolonged.

Hyperpyrexia may occur in:

1. Very severe infections;
2. Excessively hot or humid climates (heat stroke);
3. Brain stem or hypothalamic damage.

Nursing care of patients with pyrexia

The nursing care should be directed toward preventing the possible side-effects of pyrexia, the prevention and treatment of excessively high temperatures, and the administration of drugs which have been ordered.

Much of the nursing care relates directly to the excessive sweating which may occur. This sweating is a physiological adaptation which helps to reduce temperature since heat from the skin surface is used in the evaporation of sweat. The blood flowing through skin vessels is thus cooled as it circulates. Plenty of fluids should be given to replace the water lost through evaporation of sweat. The drinks should be nourishing. Electrolyte replacement may be necessary. Frequent baths and change of clothing are necessary, as is frequent mouth care. Unfortunately, the patient may have lost his appetite, but efforts should be made to maintain his energy intake, especially when pyrexia is prolonged. The temperature, pulse, respiration rates and blood pressure should be recorded frequently.

Pyrexia may be accompanied by headache, due to

intense constriction of blood vessels of the head. Photophobia and irritability may also be present. As far as possible, noise should be reduced to a minimum, bright lights should be avoided in the patient's vicinity, and the patient should be moved very gently when treatments are carried out. Analgesics may be necessary for the headache.

Measures to prevent excessively high temperatures and their treatment should they occur

1. The amount of bedclothing over the patient should be the minimum which is compatible with comfort, and the use of a bed cradle helps the circulation of air around the patient's skin surface.
2. An electric fan may be employed to cool the air around the patient. Care must be taken to ensure that the eyes are not dried excessively by the fan, especially in the case of unconscious patients.
3. Drugs which reduce temperature may be ordered by the doctor, e.g. acetylsalicylic acid, chlorpromazine, paracetamol.
4. Tepid sponging may be carried out to reduce temperature if other measures fail, or it may be used to increase the comfort of the patient.
5. In hyperpyrexia, ice packs may be used, if ordered by the doctor.

Note. Any treatment should be discontinued if shivering occurs as this will increase the body temperature.

Tepid sponging

Aims of treatment

1. To increase loss of heat from the body surface by evaporation, thus reducing body temperature.

2. The treatment should not cause shivering, since shivering causes a rise in body temperature.

Principles

1. Long sweeping strokes using a sponge soaked in tepid water leave drops of water on the skin surface, to be evaporated by the body heat.
2. Wet sponges placed in axilla and groin help to reduce the temperature.
3. A sponge which is not in use is cooled by placing it in water at a lower temperature than that being used for the procedure.
4. The temperature of the water being used for the sponge is gradually reduced during the procedure.
5. The body temperature of the patient should be recorded frequently throughout, and after the procedure, and unless specific instructions are given by the doctor, the patient's temperature should be reduced by only 1°C (2°F, approximately).

Requirements

- Supply of hot and cold water
- Bath thermometer
- Six sponges
- Face towel
- Two compresses for the forehead, soaked in iced water
- Polythene sheeting
- Two bath blankets (thin ones)
- Two large washing bowls, one containing cold water, and one containing water at the prescribed temperature; this is usually between 26° and 18°C (79° and 65°F).

Procedure

The bedclothes are removed, and the polythene sheeting and a bath blanket are rolled into position beneath the patient. The face and hands are washed and dried, and a cold compress left over the forehead. Sponges soaked in water at the prescribed initial temperature are placed in axillae and groins, and using one of the remaining sponges, the patient's arms, trunk and legs are sponged gently, leaving beads of water on the skin. Both the sponges and the cold compress must be changed from time to time, the used sponges being placed in the bowl of cold water and then transferred to the bowl of water at the correct temperature before being reused. The patient is finally turned on the side, and the back is sponged.

The procedure should take approximately 15 to 20 minutes, unless otherwise stated, and should be discontinued if the patient's temperature falls drastically, or if he complains of feeling worse.

Occasionally it may be necessary, on the doctor's instruction, to rub the skin surface whilst sponging, in order to dilate the peripheral blood vessels, since if they are constricted no evaporation of fluid by heat from the blood will take place.

At the end of the sponging, the patient should be left dry and comfortable and light clothing replaced on the bed.

THE CARE OF PATIENTS WITH HYPOTHERMIA

When people are transported to hospital with hypothermia they are usually wrapped in thermal blankets for the journey. On admission, the decision can be taken to rewarm the individual passively or actively. Since active rewarming requires medical intervention it will not be described here.

Passive rewarming includes placing the individual in a warm environment of about 25−30°C and using thermal blankets. Another method is to place the individual into a warm bath. Rewarming should be aimed at achieving an increase in core temperature of approximately 0.5°C/hour. The danger of any method of applying heat to the surface which brings about vasodilatation should be noted.

During hypothermia the metabolic rate is low. On rewarming, electrolytes and glucose may enter cells, leaving extracellular fluids depleted. Monitoring of electrolytes and blood glucose and cardiac monitoring may be carried out during rewarming.

Patients with frost-bite

Here the areas affected are rewarmed using clothing or warm water. Irreversible damage to cells is indicated by blistering, and oedematous tissue on rewarming, which changes to necrosis within about 24–48 hours. There is a danger of infection in necrotic tissue and surgery may be needed.

PART III: Special nursing problems

15 Care of the unconscious patient

Nursing an unconscious patient can be a most satisfying experience for a nurse. Nursing care can both preserve life, where death would otherwise occur, and prevent tissue damage or deformity which would severely incapacitate the patient on recovery from the coma. Caring for an unconscious patient allows the nurse to exercise to the full her skills in the physical care of people, although until such time as the patient regains consciousness, there is no use for the other skills so important in nursing, such as those of communicating with patients, and encouraging them back to independence. The nurse will, however, need to give a great deal to help and support to the relatives during this most difficult time.

An unconscious patient has lost the ability to attend to nutritional and toilet needs, together with the ability to request that these needs are attended to; the patient no longer has the ability to swallow or to control sphincter action. In deep coma, protective reflexes, such as the cough reflex and the blink reflex, are also lost. The patient is unable to change position or exercise limbs, and cannot protect himself from harmful stimuli.

There are many potential or actual nursing problems posed by unconscious patients. Nursing care is directed toward preventing these problems from occurring as well as attending to the patient's normal activities of living.

Prevention of airway obstruction

The first essential in caring for an unconscious patient is to *ensure a clear airway*, thus allowing adequate ventilation of the lungs so that the essential exchange of gases can take place between the alveolar surface and the blood. *Obstruction of the airway* may occur in several ways.

1. The tongue may be flaccid and can fall to the back of the throat.
2. Secretions from the mouth, throat or respiratory tract may accumulate in the tract itself.
3. False teeth may become displaced.
4. Vomit or regurgitation from the alimentary tract can be inhaled, causing obstruction of the airway.

To prevent obstruction of the airway, the patient may be nursed in the semi-prone or lateral position. These positions prevent the tongue from falling back, and allow vomit and excessive secretions to drain from the mouth, preventing their inhalation. Dentures should be removed from any unconscious patient, labelled and kept safely. Secretions can be removed from the back of the throat by means of gentle suction, using a sterile catheter. *Noisy respirations are signs of an obstructed airway*, and the airway must be cleared immediately.

A rubber or polythene airway may be employed to keep the tongue in position and to prevent it from falling back. It should not be employed over long periods of time, however, or ulceration of the mucous membrane will occur. If an airway of this type is employed, very frequent mouth toilet is essential, together with changing the airway and cleansing and sterilization of the used one. An endotracheal tube may be inserted to maintain the patency of the respiratory passage, but this, too, can cause ulceration of the mucosa, with stricture due to scar tissue at a later date. For this reason, it is unusual to

leave an endotracheal tube in position for longer than
48–72 hours, at which point a tracheostomy may be
performed if the breathing remains difficult. A tracheostomy not only ensures a clear airway, but it allows
secretions to be sucked out more easily, and cuts down
the ventilatory dead space, allowing better ventilation of
the lungs (see Chapter 13).

Prevention of chest infection

In the absence of the cough reflex, normal bronchial
secretions accumulate within the chest, and are very likely
to give rise to chest infection. This can be prevented by
changing the patient's position from side to side, hourly
or 2-hourly, so that each lung in turn lies uppermost,
aiding its expansion on inspiration, and draining secretions. If allowed, the foot of the bed should be raised
from time to time, further helping the secretions to drain,
and the physiotherapist should be asked to carry out
frappage to the chest wall, loosening thick mucus, which
can then be sucked from the back of the throat. The
physiotherapist should be asked to teach the correct
technique to the nursing staff, so that this treatment can
be continued at intervals throughout the 24 hours. The
physiotherapist can advise as to how frequently it should
be carried out. If chest infection does occur, in spite of
these precautions, a sputum specimen should be obtained,
so that the appropriate antibiotic can be administered to
the patient.

Artificial feeding

Since the patient is unable to swallow, an alternative
method of feeding is essential. Initially, this may be by
the intravenous route, but prolonged administration of
intravenous fluids is likely to cause thrombosis in the vein
being used. Fluids that can be administered easily by this

route do not supply the full nutritional requirements. Intragastric feeding is, therefore, the method of choice for any patient who is unconscious for any length of time. Careful checking of the tube to ensure that it is in the stomach should be carried out before each feed is given, since the tube can enter the respiratory tract without any tell-tale coughing and choking. Before each feed is given, the nurse should make sure, by aspirating the tube, that the previous feed has been absorbed or emptied from the stomach, as vomiting may occur if the stomach becomes excessively distended. The times at which the patient is turned should be calculated carefully, so that turning is carried out before intragastric feeding. Regurgitation or vomiting might occur if the patient is turned immediately after a feed. With the help of the dietitian, the feeds must be carefully calculated to give the full nutritional content and fluid requirements needed by the patient in the 24-hour period, allowing for small amounts of water to be used to clear the tube before and after each feed. The amount and frequency of each individual feed can then be determined according to the size of the patient and their individual food habits. Frequent, small, feeds may be needed for a patient who is used to small, frequent meals, whilst another patient may tolerate larger quantities, less frequently. The type of food used may need changing if the patient is not tolerating the feed well, or if diarrhoea develops (e.g. glucose and water may be absorbed better than Complan, until digestive function improves).

Sometimes unconscious patients require a higher energy content in their feeds than would be expected from their activity level. Restless patients, patients with pyrexia, or an increased metabolic rate from other causes, may lose weight whilst unconscious, unless their needs are very accurately estimated, and the energy content of their feeds increased.

In his study of the nutrition of the unconscious patient, Jones (1975) found that:

1. The diet of all 39 of the patients he observed provided less than the total energy intake recommended by DHSS.
2. All but two diets provided less than the minimum fluid requirements.
3. Diets were particularly deficient in fat and carbohydrate content.
4. Thirty-nine per cent of the diets were below the requirements recommended by Platt et al (1963) for basal metabolism.

These findings are a serious indictment of nursing care and underline the attention which should be given to prescribing the nutritional content and volume of tube feeds given to unconscious patients to maintain their body weight and hydration. Each nurse who is instructed to give a feed to an unconscious patient has a responsibility to ensure that the prescribed feed is accurately mixed and given according to instructions. The fluid chart should be completed in detail. Problems in administering the feed or poor absorption of the previous feed should be reported immediately.

A nasogastric tube should be changed daily, whilst one passed through the mouth should be removed after every feed. In general, the nasal route is more satisfactory, but the oral route should be used in head injury, nasal injury, or patients with a grossly deviated nasal septum.

Mouth toilet

Frequent mouth toilets must be carried out for an unconscious patient. Salivary secretions will not be stimulated by eating; mouth breathing is common in unconscious patients, and this not only dries the membranes, but also abolishes the changes of pressure which occur in normal breathing and stimulate the circulation of the mucous membrane. The presence of chest infection increases the need for frequent mouth cleaning, whilst a dirty mouth increases the likelihood of chest infection. Mouth toilet should be carried out 1–4-hourly.

Special precautions are required when cleaning the mouth of an unconscious patient. The swabs should be of gauze with stitched ends, so that no wisps of cotton can find their way into the respiratory system. They should be firmly clipped on to Spencer Wells forceps, and hydrogen peroxide should not be used as a cleansing agent, since it froths and could be breathed in. Petroleum jelly may be needed on the lips to prevent dryness and cracking.

Care of the skin

A daily blanket bath should be carried out, and if the patient is incontinent of urine, or perspires a lot, the bed-linen must be changed, and the skin washed and dried frequently, to prevent excoriation of the skin. Frequent turning of the patient, use of sorbo pads, and careful positioning of limbs, should prevent pressure sores from occurring. The use of an alternating pressure point mattress may be of value. When attending to the patient's needs, it is important to prevent abrasions or scratches of the skin; thus watches and rings must not be worn by the nurse, who should also place pens securely in uniform pockets so that they do not fall out. Nails should be short and smoothly filed.

Management of the bladder

It is likely that an unconscious patient will be incontinent of urine, and that the urine will endanger the skin. Wet beds may be prevented, in the case of a male patient, by placing a urinal in position, although care must be taken to prevent it from pressing on the skin. There is less chance that a urinal can be successfully used in the case of a female patient, and catheterization may be necessary to prevent bed sores. However, it is possible to prevent wet beds by placing a patient on a bedpan at frequent intervals, or by changing the bed-linen very frequently. If catheterization is carried out, great care must be taken to prevent urinary infection.

Occasionally, retention of urine may occur, and careful observation of the urinary output and the state of distension of the bladder is needed, especially if retention of urine with overflow is present. Careful recording of the estimated urinary output should be carried out by all members of staff when changing a wet bed. If retention of urine should occur, then catheterization is essential. If a self-retaining catheter is inserted, by clamping the tubing and then intermittently releasing it, 2—4-hourly, the bladder tone may be maintained. This method is preferable to open drainage for an unconscious patient.

Management of the bowel

Careful recording when the patient has a bowel action is important for observing the occurrence of diarrhoea or constipation. If severe constipation should occur, there may be some faecal overflow, simulating diarrhoea. The administration of suppositories every 2 to 3 days is a useful way of preventing constipation.

Care of the limbs

Deformity of the limbs and joints should be prevented by massage of muscles, careful positioning of limbs, and daily passive movements of all joints, through a full range of movement. A bed cradle is very useful for preventing the pressure of bedclothes upon the patient's limbs.

Care of the eyes

Since the corneal reflex may be lost, bathing of the patient's eyes should be carried out 4-hourly. If the eyelids remain open, a tarsorraphy may be necessary to prevent corneal damage by the pillow (if present) when the patient is in the semi-prone position. Corneal damage can also occur from excessive drying if the patient is being fanned for pyrexia. Half strength normal saline solution should be used for bathing the eyes. Liquid paraffin or antibiotic drops may be ordered by the doctor if the eyes become dry or infected.

Assessment of the level of consciousness

Careful observation of the patient's condition will help to establish the diagnosis, assess the effectiveness of treatment, and allow timely intervention if the patient's condition should deteriorate. Observations that should be made and recorded include assessment of the patient's conscious level. Does the patient rouse when spoken to? Obey commands? Respond to painful stimuli? The presence of any paralysis should be noted. If the patient moves limbs spontaneously, is the movement equal on each side? Is the response to painful stimuli equally brisk on either side? If brain damage is suspected, the pupillary size, equality and reaction to light should be noted. A urine specimen must be obtained on admission and tested. The blood sugar may also be estimated. Frequent recordings of temperature, pulse, respiratory rate and blood pressure will be necessary. The temperature should be recorded from the axilla or rectum, *not* orally, and particular attention must be paid to the respiratory rate; any rise or fall should be reported, since respiratory infection is such a likely complication, and in brain damage an early sign of deterioration may be change in the rhythm or rate of the respirations. The Glasgow coma scale is the most usual method of recording ongoing assessment (Figure 15.1).

The patient's relatives

Since it is difficult to estimate the exact extent to which sensory function (especially hearing) is lost by any given patient, care must be taken about what is said within the patient's hearing, and relatives should be warned about this. As with any other patient, the unconscious patient should be warned before being moved in any way. For the relatives' sake, great care should be taken with the patient's appearance, so that he looks well cared for and as attractive as possible. The hair should be regularly combed and brushed and washed at intervals if the stay in hospital is a lengthy one. Male patients should be shaved regularly.

The patient's relatives will need a great deal of information, help and support whilst the patient is unconscious, and they should be allowed to visit freely. However, if the nurse feels that it is causing them distress to be present at the bedside, less frequent visiting may be suggested, so that they reserve their strength for when the patient regains consciousness, for then he will need and appreciate their presence. If the nurse intends to suggest less frequent visiting, she should be sure that the motive is for the good of the relatives and not because the relatives are in the way, or because it is difficult or embarrassing to talk to them, and give them the help and comfort they need. Relatives should be kept informed of any change in the patient's condition, so that they can be

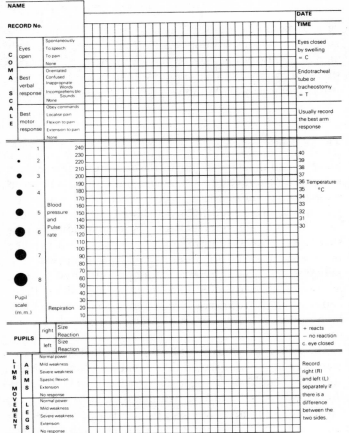

Figure 15.1 The Glasgow coma scale.

present at the bedside when the patient regains consciousness. They will also wish to be present if the patient's condition deteriorates and death is likely. It can cause them a great deal of unnecessary grief, and possible guilt, if the patient should die alone, even though he cannot be aware at the moment of dying.

16   Care of the dying

There is no doubt that the vast majority of people would prefer to go through the dying process and death in their own homes, if at all possible. Increasingly, this is adopted as the policy of health authorities. Specialist nurses, including the 'hospice at home' arrangements, can help to make care in the community a real option. However, such arrangements are not possible in every case; nor can all patients be admitted into a hospice environment. It is the care of dying patients within NHS wards that is the major concern of this chapter.

The provision of comfort for the dying is a great challenge to nursing skill, since nurses may find that their own emotional reactions to the dying patient prevent them from carrying out their role to the best of their ability. So that they may overcome these reactions, it is important that staff have insight and understanding into their origin and operation.

One common reaction to the presence of a dying patient in the ward is avoidance of that patient. On the overt level, the patient may be placed in a side room, and the staff may then avoid entering this room unless it is absolutely necessary. If the patient remains in the main ward, staff may hurry past his bed, avoiding his eye. On the other hand, a semblance of interaction may be maintained, physical needs being met and time spent in talking to the patient, but staff can still fail to give the emotional support needed, by keeping the conversation on a superficial level, talking themselves rather than letting the patient talk, evading direct questions, or giving light, flippant answers.

There are differing reasons for this avoidance reaction. Undoubtedly, caring for a dying patient can be a stressful experience. Staff may feel a sense of failure that they have not cured the patient. They may feel embarrassed at the idea of death, since death is not freely discussed in our society. To watch someone whose death is imminent can upset the onlooker, who is brought full face with a sense of his own mortality and can project himself into the situation only too easily.

A young nurse may not know how to help the patient and will feel very inadequate and inexperienced. Sometimes, inexperienced members of staff conform to the example set them, and expect that time spent with the patient just talking will gain them strong disapproval from senior staff.

Glaser and Strauss (1965) have described what they call 'awareness contexts' in relation to patients' awareness of the fact that they are dying.

'Closed awareness' is where the patient does not recognize that he is dying, even though the staff know and usually the relatives also know. The nursing problem is to prevent the patient from becoming suspicious.

'Suspicion awareness' is where the patient suspects that he is dying but does not know. Staff and relatives know. Under such circumstances, Glaser and Strauss say a verbal fencing match results in which the patient attempts to trap staff into giving away the truth. Staff have to prevent this from happening. This is one of the most difficult situations for student nurses, especially when it is the consultant's rigid policy that the patient should not be told the truth.

The patient may ask the student directly if he is dying.

The student is then faced with the dilemma of telling a lie, or being evasive, with the result of increasing or even confirming the patient's suspicions. One way of dealing with this situation is to tell the patient that the doctor is the correct person to deal with questions of that kind, and to promise to ask the doctor to come and talk to the patient. This is probably the best way in which a young inexperienced person could deal with the situation. For a more experienced person, the question could be used for getting the patient to talk and express some of his fears, which might be unrealistic and ill-founded. The nurse might therefore reply: 'What makes you ask that?' or 'What makes you think you are dying?' If the patient has good grounds for fear, again the doctor should be brought in to deal with the questions.

'Mutual pretence' occurs when the patient knows that he is dying. Staff and relatives also know, but all parties agree implicitly to pretend and to act as if the patient were going to live.

'Open awareness' is where both staff and patient know that the patient is dying and acknowledge the fact in their actions. This means that discussion about impending death can take place and the patient can be supported openly. It is the situation which usually occurs within a hospice.

THE NEEDS OF THE DYING PATIENT

A patient who knows he is dying may feel afraid of death, or may resent that this disaster has fallen on him. He may feel it is punishment for some episode in the past, or be bewildered as to why he should be singled out. The patient may feel regret that life is being cut short with things left undone, goals unachieved, opportunities lost. He may feel tired of life, and thus welcome death, or regard it as an end to pain and unhappiness.

He may simply accept the idea of death as a culmination of goals achieved, ambitions realized, or a life enjoyed to the full. More likely, feelings will vacillate between fear, resentment and acceptance.

Based on a study of over 200 dying patients, Elizabeth Kubler-Ross (1969) has described five stages through which patients who know they are dying may pass. These stages may not be of the same duration or even in the same order in all individuals. Some people will die before they have worked through the stages.

1. The first stage is '*denial with isolation*'. Denial is a defence mechanism by which we protect ourselves from anxiety when confronted with something unpleasant. This stage is often accompanied not only by feelings of isolation but by actual isolation. The patient will avoid any discussion which may force the facing of reality.

2. *Anger*. As realization of the truth is confronted, the patient feels angry to be the one singled out. This anger may spill over into verbal abuse of people with whom the patient comes into contact. Other people appear fortunate and also unable to share the patient's feelings.

3. *Bargaining*. During the stage of bargaining, the patient may feel that if only he can change his lifestyle in the future he will be saved and a cure will be found.

4. *Depression*. Depression appears to have two elements, a reaction against what has happened and anticipatory grief for what will happen in the future. Depression may be triggered by a feeling of helplessness following the patient's realization that nothing he can do will alter the outcome.

5. *Acceptance*. This is the final stage in which the patient comes to acceptance and peace. He can now talk

about what will happen with quiet confidence and make practical arrangements for his family and affairs.

Regardless of individual reactions in all except the denial stage, the patient will need to talk about his reactions and feelings and to feel free to talk about death, which, after all, is probably the most significant event of anyone's life.

A minister of religion is an ideal person to visit and listen to the patient and give him comfort. Many patients do not hold a religious belief, however, and do not wish to be visited by a chaplain. These patients particularly need to feel free to express themselves to a member of the nursing staff. Those to whom religion is important also need to be able to talk to a nurse, since the chaplain will only be able to visit infrequently.

Clinical nurse specialists or a multidisciplinary support team may counsel the patient directly, or give the benefit of their expertise to the staff caring for the patient. Support from this source can be invaluable in such a situation.

The patient needs to continue to feel a valued and useful person. He will feel valued if members of staff can spare the time to talk and to get to know him as a person. Relatives can help him to feel useful still by bringing family problems for help and advice. Unless this is done the patient will feel that no one bothers about him and he is useless. He can be helped by being brought into contemporary life as much as possible.

If it is at all possible, it is better that just one or two nurses are responsible for the patient's care, so that he can develop a close relationship with them, and not have to keep getting to know a lot of new faces. Experienced nurses rather than inexperienced should be assigned for care, since inexperienced ones may find it acutely disturbing to spend long periods of time with such a patient. The question then arises as to how they are to learn to help patients who are dying. It is impossible to teach communication skills in an abstract way. Students can best learn by listening to conversations between experienced nurses (e.g. a clinical nurse specialist), social workers, priests and the patient. Later, they can begin to talk with the patient themselves, with the situation being discussed afterwards with an experienced individual, who points out other ways in which the student could have helped the patient.

Unless the patient wishes to be in a single room, or requires such a lot of nursing care that his presence is disturbing to the other patients, it is better that he should stay in a ward with other patients to be surrounded by activity and able to participate in the ward life with the others.

Nursing care is very important to keep the patient clean and comfortable, and to help him to look as attractive as possible, maintaining both the relatives' and the patient's morale. One of the most crucial aspects of nursing care is the prompt administration of drugs prescribed by the doctor to keep the patient pain free. A great deal of the fear of dying is really a fear of pain and suffering, and the patient will be spared much anguish if confident of being kept pain free. Some patients develop the attitude when they know that they are dying that time spent by a nurse in washing or caring for him is time wasted which could be better spent on others. The nurse must make the patient feel that she enjoys giving care and attention and that he is equally as important as the other patients. Touch may begin to assume comparatively more importance than the other senses to an ill person and the nurse who can sit quietly and hold the patient's hand will help considerably. She should not feel guilty about sitting when there are other jobs to be done; and neither should she feel inadequate because she is not talking to the patient, and 'taking his mind off his troubles'.

A visit from the medical social worker may be needed so that the patient can discuss arrangements for the future of the family, and he may wish to see a solicitor or financial adviser.

SUPPORT OF RELATIVES

The patient's relatives will need continual support and advice during this time. If the patient has not been told about his imminent death, the relatives will find the situation stressful and will need to be able to discuss the situation with the doctor. They may seek advice about how to talk to the patient and how often to visit. A wife or husband may need advice on maintaining a balance between the needs of the patient and the needs of any children of the marriage. A greater dilemma will be created if relatives find the strain of visiting continually over long periods of time too much, so that their health is affected. Full and frank discussions will be needed so that both the patient and the relatives see the need to give priority to the relatives' health. The great danger is that relatives will feel both guilt and remorse, especially if the death of the patient occurs when they are not there. They must be helped to overcome these feelings of guilt, which are very normal and natural.

Discussion with the nursing staff after visiting will help relatives.

As death becomes imminent, the relatives should be notified, as well as the priest in certain religions. The relatives should be asked if they wish to stay at the hospital overnight to be present at the moment of death. If they wish to stay at home, do they want to be called in the night if there is any deterioration in the patient's condition?

Care of bereaved relatives

It often happens that death occurs of a patient who was not known to be dying, and then the notification of the relatives needs special care. Relatives should, of course, be informed of any deterioration in a patient's condition, but if they are not available, or if the patient dies suddenly, it may become necessary to inform the relatives of the fact of death with no prior preparation. If the relatives are actually present in the hospital they can be asked to sit down before the news is broken to them. Occasionally, there is no telephone number by which to contact the relatives, and a local police officer may take a message. In this case, he will ensure that the news is broken gently, and that there is someone to look after the relative before being left. A difficulty does arise if the news has to be given over the telephone to the relative who happens to be alone in the house. He should be asked to sit down before being given the news. If it is possible for the relative to fetch a neighbour this should help. It is not really practical to fetch the neighbour before the news is broken as the relative will realize something dreadful has happened and uncertainty will increase agitation. The nurse should make sure that the relative is all right before ringing off.

In the case of the sudden death of a person with religious beliefs it may be necessary to contact a representative of their faith.

The relatives should be given the opportunity of seeing the patient after death. For this visit, the patient should be made to look as peaceful as possible; the area in the vicinity of the bed should be cleared of apparatus and tidied.

If the relatives wish to see the deceased once the latter has been taken from the ward, the nursing staff can arrange for the body to be placed in the mortuary chapel and, if possible, a member of the ward staff will go with the relatives to show the way and give comfort and support.

The location of the main hospital chapel should be pointed out so that the relative may spend some time there, if wished. Tea and food should be provided as necessary.

A relative may experience shock, or feelings of guilt, and will need reassurance that everything possible was done for the patient and that the patient did not suffer at the end. An appointment should be made for the relative to see the medical social worker if advice is needed about the social agencies available to help. Before the relative leaves the hospital, the staff should see that there is someone at home on whom the relative can call for help and support. It is best if arrangements can be made for a friend or relative to spend the night with the bereaved, or to take the bereaved into their own home for the night. If there really is no one who can be called upon in this way, it might be possible to get in touch with a local health visitor or community nurse who can call in the near future to see that the bereaved relative is all right. Quite often the number of formalities to be attended to before the funeral will prevent the individual fully realizing his loss. It may only be after the funeral when the guests have all gone that the full sense of loss and grief is experienced.

There is a comparatively high incidence of depression and suicide in the period following the death of a spouse, especially amongst men. This may be associated with the modern trend for the family unit to live at a distance from relatives. In the past, and in other cultures even today, the extended family is the unit which lives together and mutual support and help in times of trouble and grief are readily available. No longer is the expression of grief allowed for by institutional ritual. Instead, it may cause friends to avoid the mourner. The period following the death of a loved one is one in which the professional support from a health visitor or social worker may help to prevent illness.

Colin Murray Parkes is a recognized authority on grief and bereavement. In a study published in 1975 he described both typical and atypical grief reactions following bereavement. It is those who undergo atypical grief reactions who are particularly at risk for psychiatric problems. Clearly, this group of people need early help if they can be identified as being at risk. Parkes found that those who suffered atypical grief reactions showed higher levels of guilt and self-reproach, delayed reaction to bereavement and prolonged grief. Experiences of loss in childhood or later, previous mental illness, or a life crisis prior to bereavement were some of the antecedent conditions that increased the risk of atypical grief. On the other hand, having social support after bereavement helped to reduce the risk of an atypical reaction.

Administrative details associated with the death

Shock may impair an individual's attention to, understanding and recall of what is said, so it is important that instructions are given to the relative very clearly, and that efforts are made to check that he has understood them. Relatives will be asked to come to the hospital to see the doctor in charge, who will be able to explain all the details of the diagnosis. The doctor may seek consent for a post-mortem examination, and will give the relative the death certificate, so that he can get on with organizing the funeral. The nursing staff should ensure that the patient's property is handed over to the relative, and a signature obtained for it. This may be done by the administrative officer of the hospital. If there should be a coroner's enquiry into the death, the coroner's officer may interview the relatives at the hospital.

LAST OFFICES

The fact that death has taken place should be certified by the medical officer. Notification of death is sent to the administrator's office. When the relatives have left the bedside, the top bedclothes are stripped from the bed, leaving a sheet covering the body. Air rings, cradles and pillows should be removed; the body should be straightened into the supine position and one pillow left under the head. The gown and any jewellery should be removed, but false teeth and the wedding ring should remain unless the relatives request otherwise. Small pledgets of damp cotton wool may be placed on the eyelids to keep them closed. The mouth should be cleaned and then closed before the jaw is bandaged into position, taking care to protect the skin from discoloration by a tight bandage by using cotton wool or plastic foam padding. If the body cannot be attended to straight away, it should be left for no longer than an hour.

Requirements

- Gown and mortuary sheet
- Washing bowl, with warm water, soap, flannel and towels
- Brush and comb. Shaving equipment in the case of a male patient
- Disposal bag for soiled dressings
- Bin for dirty linen

- A name card on which is written the patient's name, time of death, date and ward. Adhesive tape for attaching this to the mortuary sheet
- An identification band for the patient's wrist, if there is not one already in position
- Adhesive strapping
- Disposable plastic gloves
- (It may be the practice to plug the rectum and vagina with cotton wool, in which case a supply of cotton wool and disposable forceps should be available.)

Method

The body should be thoroughly washed, rinsed and dried. Nails should be cleaned, and the hair brushed out and arranged neatly. A male patient should be shaved if necessary. Any dressings should be left undisturbed. If discharge has seeped through them, fresh dressings should be placed over the existing dressings. Drainage tubes, catheters, tracheostomy tubes should be left in position. Intravenous infusion tubing should be cut near the needle insertion and strapped into position.

The gown should be put on, the body wrapped in a mortuary sheet, and the card attached to the latter with the tape, so that it can be read from the head of the patient. A nurse should supervise the lifting of the patient when the porters come to take the body to the mortuary.

All bed-linen, blankets and pillows should be sent for cleaning or washing. The bed and locker should be washed with antiseptic and dried.

The patient's possessions must be carefully packed, and checked against the list of possessions recorded on admission. Possessions acquired during the patient's stay should be added to the list, so that an accurate and up-to-date list of contents is placed with the parcel. Arrangements should be made for relatives to collect any valuables which have been placed in the safe.

THE OTHER PATIENTS

It is usual for the ward to be screened in such a way that the other patients do not get a glimpse of the dead patient, either in the ward, or during the time he is being taken to the mortuary.

If the death occurs in the daytime, it will be obvious to most patients what has happened, unless the dying patient is in a side room. When the death happens during the night, the majority of patients may be unaware that anything has happened, but they may miss the patient in the morning and enquire about him. On the whole, it is better to be frank about what has happened, since the patients may get to know the truth by other means.

17 Care of patients undergoing anaesthesia

General anaesthetics not only prevent the sensation of pain, but also abolish the natural protective reflexes. During operation, muscle relaxant drugs are usually given, and these may affect the respiratory muscles as well as the postural muscles.

The following problems may occur during or after the administration of a general anaesthetic.

- Respiratory
  Asphyxia
  Atelectasis
  Chest infection
- Cardiovascular
  Hypotension
- Alimentary
  Vomiting, or regurgitation of stomach contents
- Tissue damage
  Skin or nerve damage, due to pressure whilst the patient is unconscious.
  Deep vein thrombosis and its complication of pulmonary embolus

Surgery interrupts the continuity of tissues of the body; the skin, connective tissue, blood vessels and muscle are affected, as well as the particular organ to be operated upon. Problems which may occur include:

- Infection
- Haemorrhage, leading to shock or anaemia
- Non-healing of the wound
- Depressed activity of an organ.

Both the preoperative preparation and the postoperative care that the patient receives are directed toward preventing these problems from occurring.

PREVENTIVE MEASURES

Respiratory problems

Careful preoperative examination ensures that any pre-existing disease of the respiratory tract itself or the structures nearby can be treated. A chest X-ray will be taken, and the house surgeon or anaesthetist will listen to the chest sounds to make sure that these are normal. Any chest infection is treated with appropriate antibiotics and physiotherapy. Mouth care is important to ensure cleanliness of the mouth and teeth, and urgent dental treatment should be carried out. Any head cold or sinusitis is allowed to subside before operation is undertaken.

Postoperatively, breathing exercises are necessary, and these are usually taught preoperatively, since the patient will be in no condition to learn a new skill in the immediate postoperative period. Smoking, which irritates the mucosa, should be discouraged. Steps are taken to ensure that the stomach is empty at operation, all food and drink being withheld from the patient for 4–6 hours before the scheduled time of operation, depending on the emptying time of the stomach of the individual patient. This prevents both vomiting and excess secretion of saliva, either of which could get into the respiratory tract, whilst the cough reflex is abolished during the anaesthetic. As an extra precaution, to dry up salivary and respiratory tract secretions further, an anticholinergic drug such as atropine or hyoscine is administered by intramuscular injection 30–60 minutes before operation, along with an analgesic drug.

Asphyxia could occur during anaesthetic or immediately afterwards, due to the following:

1. The flaccid tongue falling back, obstructing the upper respiratory tract.
2. Loose dentures, displaced during the passage of the endotracheal tube or airway, may get into the upper respiratory tract. (Small plates containing one or two teeth are especially dangerous.)
3. Spasm of the vocal cords, following the removal of an endotracheal tube, can limit the air entry very considerably. If this should occur, the respirations will become very noisy with a rasping character. Immediate action is required by the anaesthetist; either the passage of an endotracheal tube or a tracheostomy may be needed.

These complications are prevented or dealt with as follows:

1. By the removal of any dentures before operation.
2. By ensuring that loose natural teeth are taken out preoperatively or, if that is impossible, that the anaesthetist knows about them.
3. When the endotracheal tube has been removed, and before the patient has regained consciousness, the tongue must be prevented from falling back. This is helped by the presence of an airway lying over the tongue and protruding through the lips and teeth, thus ensuring a free passage of air to the pharynx. To

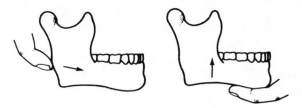

Figure 17.1 How to hold the jaw of an unconscious patient.

prevent the tongue from falling back if the patient is lying in a recumbent position, the jaw should be held up and forward (Figure 17.1). If possible, the patient should lie in a semi-prone position; this will both prevent the tongue from falling back and help any vomit or excessive secretions to run out of the mouth, rather than back into the respiratory passages.

4. The character of the respirations should be observed carefully and, if laryngeal spasm occurs, oxygen should be given until the anaesthetist arrives, an immediate message having been delivered to him. Another nurse can be collecting together the equipment for intubation, so that it is available.

5. If the face shows any cyanosis, the patient will need oxygen, so colour should be observed. Whenever oxygen is to be given, the first essential is to ensure a clear airway (i.e. a clear respiratory tract). A high concentration of oxygen in the air available for inspiration is useless unless it can get to the alveolar membrane for exchange with the blood gases.

6. 'Anaesthetic instruments', which are useful in any respiratory emergency, should accompany the patient to the operating theatre, so that they are available during the journey back to the ward. These instruments are: tongue depressor, tongue clips, mouth gag,

and gauze swabs (with bound edges) clipped firmly into sponge-holding forceps. Using these instruments, it is possible to open the mouth of the patient, pull the tongue forward, and remove any secretions accumulating in the back of the throat.

Postoperatively, the important thing is to encourage full inflation of the lungs, so the patient is put into a sitting position allowing good descent of the diaphragm as soon as the condition will allow. Deep breathing exercises are encouraged shortly after operation. If necessary, expectoration is aided by the use of inhalations, physiotherapy to the chest wall and postural drainage. The patient's temperature and respiratory rates are recorded to detect the onset of chest infection, so that antibiotics may be started and vigorous treatment instituted. If the throat has been sprayed during the operation, fluids and food must be withheld until the effects of the anaesthetic spray have worn off. Postoperative vomiting should be prevented by cautiously reintroducing foods and fluids, and the use of antiemetic drugs, if necessary.

Cardiovascular problems

Pre-existing cardiovascular disease could endanger the patient during the operation. Thus, careful examination of the cardiovascular system is part of the preparation for operation; special attention being paid to the functioning of the heart, the blood pressure, and the haemoglobin content of the blood. A preoperative course of digoxin may be necessary in elderly patients and, if the haemoglobin level is below normal, this will need correction, probably by transfusion before operation. Blood is routinely grouped and cross-matched before any but the most minor of operations, and blood is ordered in the quantity appropriate to the expected blood loss at operation. The patient's pulse and blood pressure should be recorded by the nursing staff preoperatively to provide a comparison for the postoperative recordings. This is especially important for a hypertensive patient in whom a blood pressure of, say, 120 mmHg systolic may appear normal, unless a preoperative record is available, when it is revealed to be very low for that particular patient.

Many drugs which are given to individuals over a long period of time can cause cardiovascular disturbances, either by potentiation of drugs given during anaesthesia, or because they are withdrawn suddenly before anaesthesia. The anaesthetist should be aware of all medication that the patient has been receiving, so that suitable precautions may be taken. Drugs which may affect the cardiovascular system in either of these ways include corticosteroids, whose sudden withdrawal may be associated with hypotension; monoamine oxidase inhibitors, whose presence may cause either hypertension or hypotension; diuretics, which can cause severe hypotension; and antihypertensive drugs, which can also cause hypotension.

Careful postoperative observation of the patient is necessary to detect the early signs of shock, shown by an increasing pulse rate, a low blood pressure, restlessness or an increasing pallor. Shock may arise as a result of bleeding, and the dressings covering the wound should be carefully observed for this. The only satisfactory treatment of shock is to increase the circulating blood volume by the intravenous administration of fluid. Any bleeding, of course, must be stopped, and the legs should be raised to form an angle of about 45° with the trunk. This allows the increased return of venous blood from the lower limbs to the heart, increasing cardiac output.

If a blood transfusion is in progress when the patient returns from the operating theatre, careful observation of the body temperature to detect an incompatibility reaction is necessary, together with careful recording of the pulse rate, the rate of infusion, and inspection of the infusion site to ensure that it is not running subcutaneously. Similar observations will be necessary if the patient is receiving an infusion of fluid other than blood. A fluid intake and output record will be needed if the patient is receiving intravenous fluid, to ensure that the vascular compartment is not being overloaded; in any case, careful observation of the urinary output is necessary, since kidney damage and anuria can result from a low blood pressure.

The risk of deep vein thrombosis is increased by operation, partly due to increased blood viscosity after tissue damage during surgery, and partly due to the slowing of the venous flow in the calf veins and compression whilst the patient is on the operating table. Thus, lower limb exercise should be encouraged very early after operation, and the patient is allowed out of bed for bedmaking, as soon as possible. Antiembolic stockings of the correct size, correctly worn and applied preoperatively may be very useful in preventing deep vein thrombosis. A slight rise in temperature and/or pulse rate may be the first clue that this complication has occurred. Anticoagulation may then be necessary to prevent a pulmonary embolus.

Wound infection and delayed healing

The patient will be carefully examined for the presence of any infective lesion before operation and, if possible, the operation should be delayed until the patient is infection free. A course of antibiotics may be started preoperatively. The patient should be as healthy as possible, before and after operation, to promote resistance to infective organisms, so a good nutritious diet should be given; high protein or vitamin supplements may be necessary.

Before operation, the skin at the operation site and for a wide surrounding area should be shaved clear of hairs, which are a source of microorganisms, especially of staphylococci. The patient should then have a bath; further preparation of the skin by painting with an antiseptic lotion may be carried out in the ward, but in any case will be carried out in the operating theatre before the incision is made. If collection of body fluids or stale blood within the wound is foreseen, either of which could exert pressure upon the suture line or act as a focus for inflammation, delaying healing, the surgeon will insert a drain before closing the wound. Stitches or clips are used to keep the wound edges in apposition to one another; the amount of regenerated tissue needed to fill the gap is thus kept at a minimum and healing takes place rapidly (by 'first intention').

Clean blankets are used to cover the patient when taken from the ward to the operating theatre; thus there is a reduced possibility of carrying microorganisms from the ward to the threatre. Whilst the patient is being operated on, the bed is cleaned and remade with clean linen into a 'pack' ready for his return. The use of clean linen helps to prevent the contamination of the dressings with microorganisms.

Postoperatively, the wound should be kept clean, by means of dressings. It should be uncovered only when absolutely necessary. As soon as possible, the drains and stitches are removed, using an aseptic, atraumatic technique; the longer these are left in position, the greater the chance that they will initiate an inflammatory reaction, since they are 'foreign' to the patient's tissue, yet they must remain long enough to allow healing to take place. The interval for which the stitches or clips are left in position depends on two factors: (1) the site of operation, e.g. the scalp heals very rapidly and stitches can be removed within 48 hours of operation, whilst the stitches following laminectomy will be removed only after 10 to 14 days; and (2) the rapidity with which the individual patient's skin heals. Healing may be delayed if there is a poor blood supply to the area, or if in the presence of infection. The prevention of postoperative shock will help to maintain a good blood supply to the area. Careful observation and the judicious use of intravenous fluids will thus be necessary. It is important to observe for signs or symptoms of wound infection. Pain, throbbing or local heat in the area may be the symptoms complained of by the patient, whilst redness of the area or pyrexia will indicate the presence of infection.

Prevention of damage of the patient

The patient is unconscious during the administration of a general anaesthetic, and therefore unable to care for himself in any way. Normal protective reflexes are abolished, and the hospital staff must ensure that he comes to no harm in this time. Some means of identification must be attached to the patient, e.g. by a wristband; the skin should be marked on the side of operation when operation is planned on one of paired organs; these measures ensure that only the operation needed by the patient is carried out. Notes, X-rays, and prescription sheet should accompany the patient to the operating theatre.

Before the operation is carried out, the patient must have given written consent. In the case of a minor, or an unconscious patient, the next of kin is asked to sign the operation consent form. Immediately before operation, anything that could cause damage by pressure or in the presence of diathermy is removed from the person of the patient, including hairgrips and all jewellery except the wedding ring which is covered with adhesive tape to prevent it slipping off the finger. An operating gown which is secured by tapes is substituted for the patient's own night attire. Great care must be taken to prevent nerve damage whilst the patient is unconscious; positioning of limbs must be done with care. The eyes must be protected by the lids, to prevent corneal damage, and the patient's hair should be covered by a cotton turban, so that there is no risk of it getting into the eyes.

Pain

Preoperatively, an analgesic such as morphine, Omnopon, pethidine or pentazocine is administered by injection, together with the anticholinergic drug. There are several reasons for the administration of a drug of this type. As such drugs are sedative in action as well as analgesic, they ensure that the patient is in a calm sleepy condition when he goes to the operating theatre. The drug also helps to prevent immediate postoperative pain. Further analgesia will be needed postoperatively when its effects have worn off. Ideally, the patient should be kept pain free. Pain is very unpleasant, and it will curtail movement, possibly affecting the respirations. If the wound is in the abdominal or chest area, the respirations may become very shallow and the patient will be unable to cough or expectorate in the presence of pain. It can be seen how other complications may occur if pain is not adequately treated.

A patient who is nursed in a small room rather than in an open ward may need special observation to ensure that he obtains the analgesics needed. Patients in small rooms may feel reluctant to call a nurse. Some patients feel uncomfortable at the idea of ringing for a nurse because 'I know the nurses are busy'. It was found that patients in a ward divided into small bedded units were given only about half the postoperative analgesia received by a comparable group of patients in an open ward (Hayward, 1975). Furthermore, in an open ward a patient may emit 'cues' which can be recognized and acted upon by a nurse who may be engaged in an entirely different task.

Since Hayward's study, a great deal of further research knowledge about pain is available. This includes knowledge of people's pain experience and of methods of intervention to alleviate pain (McCaffery, 1979). In relation to postoperative care, the type of pain which will be experienced is acute pain, whilst it is chronic pain which is particularly problematic in terms of management. None the less, we do know that expecting patients to report pain and ask for analgesia is an inadequate method of managing their pain. Under such circumstances the patient will suffer both whilst waiting to catch the nurse's attention, and during the interval whilst the drug is obtained and administered. It also takes time before the drug begins to exert its effects.

The aim of nursing intervention should be to keep the patient pain free. This means administering drugs promptly at the intervals allowed by the prescription, even if the patient is pain free at the time. It also means that the patient's pain level should be assessed 30–45 minutes after the drug was administered to assess its effectiveness. If the patient is not pain free, then the doctor should be asked to prescribe a larger dose or a more effective drug. Pain assessment may be carried out using a simple visual analogue scale such as one shown in Figure 17.2. Relaxation and other similar techniques (see McCaffery, 1979) can be taught to the patient as ways of helping to relieve pain. Such techniques are particularly useful because they give the patient a strategy to use whenever pain is experienced, thus giving a measure of control. It is important

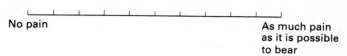

Figure 17.2 Analogue scale for recording pain. In practice the line would measure 10 cm.

to remember McCaffery's definition of pain whenever pain management is needed: 'Pain is whatever the patient says it is, and exists when he says it does.'

Hayward's study also suggested that the major influence upon the amount of analgesic received by patients postoperatively was the policy of the nursing staff concerned. This is interesting since drugs are prescribed by the doctor. It seems that the doctor's prescription sets the limits within which the day-to-day decisions about administration of drugs are made by nurses. This places a responsibility upon nurses to ensure that individual differences of patients in both their need for analgesics and their response to them are met by individual observation and care. It is not enough to have set routines of analgesic administration based upon the type of operation or, worse still, as a ward routine. Sometimes nurses become unnecessarily worried about the dangers of narcotic and analgesic drugs. The administration of such drugs to relieve pain during the relatively short time in which pain occurs postoperatively is unlikely to cause dependence. Generally, as the patient recovers, the need for drugs disappears rapidly.

Alimentary tract problems

Peristalsis ceases during the general anaesthetic, and the stomach is empty at the time of operation. The return to a full diet should proceed gradually, or vomiting may occur. Sips of water only are given in the immediate postoperative period, then a light diet, and usually not until the first postoperative day or later does the patient return to a full diet. One cannot lay down any hard and fast rules about this; however, the site and severity of the operation must be taken into account, as well as the reaction of the individual patient.

Constipation may occur postoperatively as a result of the administration of morphine, lack of exercise, lack of solid food, or a change in diet. Aperients or suppositories may be necessary if the patient's normal pattern of bowel action is grossly upset.

Flatus, accumulating in the bowel, may be extremely uncomfortable for the patient. A flatus tube passed via the anus will usually relieve this satisfactorily.

Complications of the alimentary tract are most likely to occur when the operation is on the tract itself, or in its vicinity (e.g. gynaecological operations). Prolonged administration of drugs such as morphine, which depress peristalsis, can also give rise to complications of the tract. The main danger is of cessation of peristalsis, with accumulation of fluids or gas within the tract causing gross distension. This is prevented in high risk patients by keeping the alimentary tract empty in the immediate postoperative period. A nasogastric tube is passed immediately before operation, and either continuous or intermittent gentle suction keeps the stomach empty after operation. Carefully measured sips of water may be allowed postoperatively but an intravenous infusion is maintained until bowel sounds are heard. A fluid balance chart must be kept. If paralytic ileus should arise as a postoperative complication, it is treated by the passage of a nasogastric tube, stomach aspiration and an intravenous infusion. Antibiotics are usually given.

Urinary tract problems

The urine of every patient is tested on admission to hospital, and the result of that test usually accompanies the patient to theatre. It is important that not only metabolic disorders such as diabetes mellitus are revealed by urine testing, but that abnormalities of the urinary system itself are detected. In an elderly patient, the blood urea may be estimated.

Immediately before the operation the patient should empty the bladder, but if the operation is to be carried out on the bladder or in its vicinity (e.g. gynaecological operations), a self-retaining catheter is inserted and the bladder is drained.

A sustained low blood pressure affects the renal blood flow, and anuria may result. Shock must, therefore, be prevented and careful observation will ensure that , should it occur, it is detected very early and can be treated before any renal damage occurs. If the blood pressure was low during operation, a fluid balance chart should be recorded postoperatively. If anuria does occur, then a self-retaining catheter will be inserted to allow the urinary output to be recorded accurately. Fluid and dietary restriction, peritoneal dialysis, or an artifical kidney will be necessary until kidney function returns.

If a patient does not pass urine postoperatively, it may be due to retention of urine or anuria, and it is important to observe for both these condtions and to distinguish between them. Thus, careful observation and reporting when the patient micturates postoperatively will save a lot of anxiety. If the patient fails to pass urine within about 18 hours of operation, the fact should be reported so that the bladder may be examined. If it should be distended, then he may be allowed to stand (male patient) or use a commode (female patient) in the hope that a more natural position will help. An injection of carbachol (0.2–0.5 mg) may be needed to relax the urethral sphincter but, since this substance has unpleasant side-effects, catheterization may be preferred. The patient will usually be able to pass urine later, when more mobile.

PSYCHOLOGICAL EFFECTS

If the patient is to have complete faith in the surgeon who is carrying out the operation, full explanation must be given of the diagnosis and the operation necessary to relieve the condition. The patient must have complete trust in the surgeon to put himself at the surgeon's mercy whilst unconscious and unable to know what is happening. If there is the slightest doubt of the diagnosis, the possibility of a more radical operation than the planned operation should be mentioned, since if the patient recovers from the anaesthetic to find that he has lost a greater amount of the body than expected, this can have a profound effect, causing acute depression and lack of trust in the hospital staff. This in turn could delay physical recovery. The operation consent form usually includes a clause to cover this eventuality, but not all patients read the form carefully before signing. Their attention should be drawn to this clause, and steps should be taken to ensure that the patient has fully understood the implications.

As with everything else that is done in hospital, the way in which the preparation, the operation itself, and the postoperative care will affect the patient must be carefully explained. The reduction of uncertainty thus afforded will not only help the patient's subjective feelings, but adequate explanation related to specific aspects of the effects of operation actually reduces the incidence of postoperative complications which occur. The account by Hayward (1975) of his interviews of 40 postoperative patients deserves particular attention. His results indicate areas in which careful explanation must become part of the nursing preparation of patients undergoing operation.

Of his sample of patients, 70% found that one or more aspect of anaesthesia caused anxiety. A particular concern was their lack of knowledge of how the anaesthetic would be given and elderly patients, especially, worried that it would be given by face mask.

The preoperative procedure should be explained to patients beforehand and the reason for each procedure must be explained. Several of the patients interviewed found that shaving, donning gowns and waiting in isolation behind curtains was stressful and they felt very lonely and depersonalized.

Very careful explanation of the premedication injection is needed as some patients confused this with the anaesthetic and were alarmed that the expected effect of an anaesthetic did not occur following the injection.

Of the patients interviewed, 35% had been taken by surprise by the severity of the postoperative pain. This was particularly the case with the younger patients, some of whom were resentful about the apparent lack of information on this subject.

About 60% of the patients did not understand the therapeutic reason for getting them out of bed soon after operation and thought it was for the nurses' convenience.

Many patients expect to regain consciousness in their beds in the same spot of the ward which they occupied preoperatively. If they are to be nursed in a recovery room or in a different ward position postoperatively, this must be explained preoperatively.

Other things which cause concern if the individual is unprepared are infusions and drainage tubes. Many of these points will be explained by the doctor. This does not absolve the nurse from responsibility though, as so often the doctor uses language which is not easily understood by the patient.

Hayward went on to carry out an experiment in which a group of patients received information about the preoperative and postoperative procedures and the pain and discomfort which might occur. A comparable group of patients was engaged in conversation which conveyed no specific information for the exact period of time it took to give the information to the first group of patients. Results showed that the patients receiving information required less analgesia postoperatively than the uninformed group. Morale and measures of comfort also showed the beneficial effects of the information upon the group of patients receiving it.

Since Hayward's study there have been many other experimental studies of this type carried out both in this country and in the USA. As a result of such studies, benefits of preoperative information upon all dimensions of postoperative recovery have been confirmed. Indeed researchers in the USA (Devine and Cook, 1986) have concluded that a net saving of $100 per patient per operation occurs due to more rapid recovery, balanced against the time spent in giving preoperative information. Various types of preoperative information have been evaluated for their effectiveness. These can be classified as:

1. *Procedural information.* This is information about what will be done, in what order, and approximately how long different elements of the procedure will take.
2. *Sensory information.* Here the emphasis is on how the patient will experience the events which occur. This information should include details of the pain likely to be experienced, any nausea, faintness and discomfort.

In addition, any unusual sights, sounds, tastes or smells associated with the experience are explained.

3. *Behavioural instruction*. This is informational teaching about what the patient needs to do to help the professional carrying out the procedure, or to help themselves. Breathing exercises, leg exercises and relaxation techniques are examples of behaviour which can be taught preoperatively.

4. *Cognitive instruction*. This is information which encourages the patient to think about things in a different and positive way. The technique can help to lower anxiety levels. For example, patients are taught to think of the benefits which will accrue from operation in terms of improved health, mobility, etc. Distraction by thinking of pleasant and positive events is also taught.

Research has shown that the information which is the most effective in terms of postoperative recovery is the sensory information. It is difficult to give sensory information alone, however, since procedural information is also needed to make sense of the sensory information.

A small number of patients have been found not to benefit from preoperative information. Therefore, very careful assessment of the patient's information needs and preferred coping style is required. Those patients who are found on assessment to be unlikely to benefit from information should be given emotional support instead.

In general, the underlying principle in giving information is that it helps the patient to plan and develop coping strategies and it also helps the patient's feelings of being in control. This helps to reduce excessive anxiety and stress levels. Information-giving requires an individual approach catered to the patient and his needs. Time and repetition of information are necessary. High anxiety levels interfere with the retention of information. Clearly, information that is not remembered cannot help the patient cope. Thus, the way in which a nurse is able to reduce the anxiety levels of a patient through giving information is a valuable measure of nursing skill.

18   Assessment and monitoring

Assessment of the patient is not just something that is carried out on admission, but it continues throughout the stay in hospital. Assessment includes the evaluation of the outcome of nursing care.

Specific observations of the patient's condition are also carried out by nursing staff in order to help the medical staff to monitor the patient's condition or even to establish the diagnosis.

There is always a nurse on duty in a ward, whereas the doctor only visits at intervals. Between visits doctors rely on the nursing staff to keep them informed of any deterioration in the patient's condition which might require surgical intervention, a change of treatment, or even resuscitation of the patient. To carry out this nursing function adequately, the nurse must observe the patient, keep records of the observations, interpret them, and make a decision as to whether or not any action is required.

Proper *observation* of the patient requires not only that the nurse should observe the patient's conscious level, colour, temperature, pulse rate, respiration and blood pressure at intervals as required, but also whilst working in the ward remaining receptive, or sensitive to stimuli emitted by her patients. Thus the nurse notices a change in the respiratory rhythm of a patient whose respirations are noisy, even though it occurs in the interval between formal observations. Similarly she notices that a patient has become restless, or is in pain, even whilst merely walking past the patient's bed to attend to someone else.

Each nurse is off duty for approximately 16 out of 24 hours. It is important, therefore, that observations made of patients are accurately *communicated* from the nurse making the observation to other members of staff. Written *records* are kept of many of the observations that are made. These aid communication, ensure continuity of care, and provide a permanent record of the condition of the patient over a period of time.

Interpretation of observations that are made requires two kinds of knowledge. Firstly, a knowledge of how this observation compares with the normal value for the population of which the patient is a member, and secondly, a knowledge of how this observation compares with the normal values for this particular patient. For instance, to interpret the significance of a patient's pulse rate one needs to know not only the normal pulse rate for people of the patient's age group and activity, but also to know the patient's previous pulse rate. The normal or average pulse rate of an adult at rest is 72/minute. A pulse rate of 50/minute would cause disquiet if observed in a patient with an intracranial lesion, whose previous pulse rate was higher than this. It could, however, be the normal rate for a trained athlete, and would merely reflect a physiological adaptation. A pulse rate rising to 80/minute in the trained athlete at rest should be investigated further however, although it would be considered normal if one had no previous recording with which to compare it.

An observation of a single bodily function, although better than nothing, gives little information, and the greater the number of different functions assessed at the same time, the more pieces of evidence are obtained to allow correct interpretation. A pulse rate of 50/minute is of no special significance in an individual who looks healthy, is alert mentally, is active physically, and whose blood pressure, temperature and respiratory rate are normal. The same pulse rate in an individual who is very drowsy, who is developing some paralysis, and whose blood pressure is rising, should cause concern.

Thus, interpretation of individual observations depends upon comparison with the normal for a given group of individuals, a knowledge of the result of previous observations of this particular patient, and the sum total of observations on several different parameters at the time of the present observation.

The interpretation of any given sign or symptoms involves a *decision*, as to its significance in the light of the nurse's knowledge (Figure 18.1). This decision determines whether or not the nurse must take immediate resuscitative action whilst getting a message to the doctor, whether to inform the doctor of the patient's condition but take no other action for the moment, whether to wait but observe

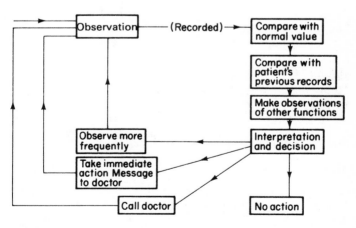

Figure 18.1   Flow diagram of observation-decision process.

the patient more frequently, or whether no action is required.

TEMPERATURE AND ITS MEASUREMENT

The temperature of a body is a measure of its warmth or coldness compared with a standard, such as boiling or freezing water. On the Celsius scale the boiling point of pure water at standard atmosphere pressure (760 mmHg) is marked as 100°C (212°F), and the freezing point as 0°C (32°F). The scale between these points is divided into 100; thus each degree Celsius is a measure of 1/100th of the difference between the heat energy of boiling water and freezing water. A thermometer, used to record temperature, is based on the principle that matter expands on heating and contracts on cooling, and it is constructed so that coloured liquid of some kind, held in a reservoir, can only expand along a narrow glass stem which is marked with an appropriate scale to indicate temperature. Measurement of the temperature of the human body is carried out using a clinical thermometer, which most frequently has mercury in its bulb. In the stem immediately above this is a constriction which causes a break in the thread of the mercury when the thermometer is removed from contact with the body. Thus it remains at the level of temperature reached whilst it was in equilibrium with the body temperature and can be read. It must be shaken down each time before a new temperature is recorded.

Body temperature

The healthy human body, far from reflecting the temperature of the environment, remains within rather narrow limits of 35.5–37.2°C (96–99°F). This narrow range of temperature is maintained by a controlling system of cells in the hypothalamus. Mechanisms for conserving, producing or losing heat are brought into use according to the temperature of the blood circulating through the hypothalamic heat centre, together with less important information from temperature receptors in the skin.

Both muscular and metabolic activities of the body produce heat energy as a side-product, and this heat is dispersed rapidly throughout the body by means of the bloodstream. Vascular changes at the skin surface help in the control of body temperature, heat conservation being increased by the constriction of the blood vessels which reduces the flow of the blood through the skin; whilst heat loss is increased by the dilatation of peripheral blood vessels. The greater blood flow which results allows loss of heat, not only by radiation and conduction, but also by evaporation of sweat. Heat is lost unavoidably in expired air and in excreta. Control of temperature in infants and the aged is less efficient than in children and adults.

Normally, there is a diurnal variation in body temperature, the temperature being higher in the evening and lower in the morning.

Pyrexia is the term denoting a body temperature raised above the normal range, and this may occur either if the metabolic rate is increased or if the hypothalamic centre is affected by 'pyrogens' from microorganisms or broken down tissue cells.

Hyperpyrexia is used to describe a body temperature of 40°C (104°F) or more. A patient with a body temperature above normal may be said to have a *fever*. Terms such as continuous fever, remittent fever (an exaggeration of diurnal variation), intermittent fever (where pyrexia and normal temperature alternate but less frequently than diurnally), have been used to described the patterns seen on the temperature charts of patients with particular types of infection. Antibiotics usually suppress these patterns today. *Crisis* was a term used to describe the sudden drop of temperature to normal levels within a few hours after severe fever. During a crisis the heat loss is greater than heat production.

Hypothermia is the term used for a state where the body temperature is below the normal range, and it may accompany shock, or be brought about by prolonged exposure to cold, or to cold, wet, windy conditions. It also accompanies an excessively low metabolic rate.

Any deviation of the patient's temperature from normal should be reported. Particular care should be taken when recording the temperature of patients who might be suffering from hypothermia, since the usual clinical thermometer does not record subnormal temperature, and a special thermometer may be needed.

To record the patient's temperature

Principles

1. A clinical thermometer is reserved for the individual use of the patient throughout the hospital stay, and/or is sterilized each time it is used.
2. It should be dried before use, and the mercury should be shaken below the markings on the thermometer.
3. It should be placed in the selected position and left there for a minimum of 6 minutes and preferably for 9 minutes before being removed and read.
4. Care should be taken that the temperature recorded by the thermometer is not affected by conditions peculiar to the particular area used to take the temperature, so that the temperature as recorded is an accurate reflection of the core temperature.

Requirements

- The patient's clinical thermometer
- Swabs for drying the thermometer before use
- Disposal bag for used swabs
- A watch with a second hand
- The patient's temperature chart and a pen
- Petroleum jelly if the rectal temperature is to be recorded

Areas which may be selected for recording the temperature

The mouth. This is the most commonly used area for taking the patient's temperature, but there are many situations and conditions in which it is best to avoid using the mouth; these include: if the patient has recently swallowed hot or cold fluid or food; if he cannot close the mouth for any reason; if breathing is difficult or rapid; if the mouth is inflamed or sore; or if he is confused, or comatose. Oral temperatures should not be recorded in infants and young children.

The patient is asked to hold the thermometer under the tongue, closing the lips but not the teeth. He should be requested not to talk whilst the thermometer is in position.

The axilla or groin. Recording the temperature from the axilla or groin should be avoided in patients who are very thin so that two skin surfaces cannot be in contact with the thermometer at the same time. It will not reflect core temperature in a patient who is in a state of shock, or whose peripheral blood vessels are constricted for any other reason. The skin surfaces must be dry whilst the thermometer is in position.

The rectum. It can be very embarrassing for a patient to

have the temperature recorded per rectum; therefore, other methods should be used if possible. Rectal temperatures are sometimes recorded in babies and young infants whilst they are being bathed or having their nappies changed.

To record a baby's temperature, he is placed, lying on the back, on the nurse's knee, with the hips flexed and the knees straight so that the legs are at angle of 90° to the body. The lubricated thermometer is then passed through the anus for about 1.3 cm and held in position by the nurse, who holds the legs in position with the other hand.

For adults, the procedure must be carefully explained, and the thermometer is lubricated with petroleum jelly before use. The patient should be in the lateral position with knees and hips flexed, and the thermometer should be held in position by the nurse. It is inserted through the anus about 3.5 cm.

When the thermometer has been in position for a minimum of 6 minutes, and preferably for 9 minutes, it is withdrawn, the temperature is read, and the thermometer is returned to an antiseptic solution, so that it is disinfected before being shaken down. The temperature should be charted.

Sometimes very accurate or frequent records of 'core' temperatures are required. An electronic thermometer may be used, the lead of which is placed into the oesophagus or rectum and left in position. The machine is then switched on to record the temperature.

THE PULSE

A pulse is the wave of expansion felt in artery walls when the heart pumps blood into the aorta which, because it contains elastic tissue in its wall, is thus distensible. This distension, when the aorta accommodates the blood from the left ventricle, spreads rapidly along the walls of the whole arterial system, but dies out before reaching the capillaries. A pulse can be felt wherever a superficial artery runs over a bone, e.g. radial, facial, temporal, posterior tibial and dorsalis pedis arteries. Pulsation can also be felt in the carotid arteries in the neck.

In normal individuals, the pulse rate accurately reflects the heart rate, and is recorded mainly as an indication of heart rate. Pulses may also be recorded at the extremities, especially in the lower limbs, to observe the adequacy of the blood supply to distal parts when there is disease of the arteries.

The normal pulse rate of a resting, healthy individual varies with age. In infancy it is 120−140/minute; at 3 years of age it falls to about 100/minute, whilst the average rate for an adult is 72/minute. In old age, the rate slows further. For adults, rates between 50 and 90/minute can be regarded as within normal limits, although a pulse rate of 50 in a patient whose pulse is normally 90, and vice versa, requires investigation. Exercise and emotion, e.g. anxiety, as on admission of a patient, both increase the heart rate above the resting values quoted.

Disorders of heart rate

Recordings of the pulse rate are made to detect changes in the heart rate associated with disease, or changes in the patient's condition.

Tachycardia is the term used to denote an increase in heart rate. This may occur in the following conditions.

1. Pyrexia, and its accompanying increased metabolic rate. The heart rate increases by 10 beats/minute for every 0.5°C (1°F) rise in body temperature above normal.
2. Increased metabolic rate due to thyrotoxicosis.

3. A decrease in the effective criculating blood volume (shock).
4. Heart muscle which is failing.
5. Nervous disorder of the heart beat, called paroxysmal tachycardia.
6. Due to some drugs, e.g. atropine, amyl nitrite.

Bradycardia refers to a heart rate which is slower than normal, and this may be associated with the following conditions.

1. Excessive stimulation of the vagus nerve, as when the vagal nucleus is compressed due to increased intracranial pressure.
2. Disease of the conducting tissue of the heart, leading to 'heart block' where the ventricles contract at their own intrinsic rate.
3. When the metabolic rate is decreased, as in myxoedema.
4. When excessive amounts of digitalis are given. Not only slowing of the heart rate but also coupling may occur in which two beats of unequal force are followed by an extra long pause in a regular pattern. The pulse rate and rhythm should always be checked immediately before giving a dose of digitalis, and the presence of coupled beats, or a pulse rate of 60/minute or less, should be reported, and the dose then omitted until medical orders have been given.

Disorders of the rhythm of the heart beat

The heart beat is normally regular in rhythm except that occasionally the condition of *sinus arrhythmia* may be present, especially in children and young adults. In sinus arrhythmia the heart rate increases on inspiration and decreases on expiration; it is physiological and of no pathological significance. Whenever the pulse rate is being counted the rhythm should also be noted, and if it is irregular the pulse rate should be counted for a whole minute. In this case the apex beat should also be counted simultaneously by a second person using a stethoscope, and both rates recorded on the chart. Any irregularities in the strength of the beat should also be noted.

Extrasystole is a condition in which an extra beat of the ventricles of the heart follows rapidly on the previous beat and is followed by an abnormally long pause. The patient may be aware of this and it may cause some anxiety since subjectively it seems as if the heart 'stops'. In young people extrasystole is often associated with excessive smoking, strong coffee, fatigue or a septic focus. In an older individual it may indicate some damage to the heart muscle.

Atrial fibrillation

Fibrillation occurs when the atrial muscle no longer contracts as a whole, and a series of small and inadequate contractions pass over the muscle at a rapid rate, only some of these stimulating the ventricular muscle. Not all of the ventricular contractions eject sufficient blood to be reflected in the arterial pulses, thus the ventricular contraction rate will be greater than the pulse rate, the difference between the two being known as the pulse deficit. Atrial fibrillation may occur in mitral stenosis, coronary heart disease and thyrotoxicosis.

Recording the pulse rate

The pulse rate may be counted wherever a superficial artery runs over a bone and also at the carotid artery in the neck; the radial and temporal arteries are the most convenient. The patient should have been resting for

15 minutes and the arm should be in a comfortable position, either at the side or, more conveniently, palm down across the chest. This latter position allows respirations to be counted either immediately before or immediately after the pulse rate is counted, whilst the nurse appears to be recording the pulse rate. By this means an alteration in the respiratory rate or rhythm due to self-consciousness on the part of the patient may be prevented.

To record the pulse, the nurse's fingers should be placed along the course of the radial artery on the thumb side of the anterior surface of the wrist. The nurse should observe the regularity of rhythm and the force of the pulse before beginning to count the rate. The arterial pulsations must be counted for a minimum of half a minute and the result doubled. If there is any irregularity present, the pulsations must be counted for a minute or the rate will be recorded inaccurately.

BLOOD PRESSURE

Blood pressure is the pressure exerted by the blood upon the walls of the blood vessels. It is usually recorded in the arteries, where it is greater during the contraction of the ventricles (systolic pressure) than during the period in which the heart is relaxed (diastolic pressure).

Arterial blood pressure depends upon several factors.

1. The force of the ventricular contractions.
2. The heart rate.
3. The quantity of blood returned to the heart.
4. Resistance to blood flow in the arterioles. (If the plain muscle in the walls of these vessels contracts, then the calibre of the vessels decreases, the resistance to blood flow increases, and so does the arterial blood pressure.)
5. The state of the arterial walls. If their normal disten-

sible state, associated with the elastic fibres, is lost, then there is an increase in arterial blood pressure.

6. The quantity of effectively circulating blood. An increase in this volume causes an increase of blood pressure, whilst a reduction causes a low blood pressure, unless homeostatic mechanisms compensate effectively.

7. The viscosity of the blood.

Note. The force of the ventricular contraction, the quantity of blood returned to the heart and the heart rate together determine the *cardiac output* in terms of amount of blood per minute.

Blood pressure is recorded in millimetres of mercury (mmHg) and the normal arterial systolic pressure of a healthy adult at rest is sufficient to support a column of mercury 120 mm in height. Thus, normal arterial systolic blood pressure is quoted as 120 mmHg whilst the average arterial diastolic pressure of an adult at rest is 80 mmHg. Blood pressure tends to rise with age, so average arterial systolic pressure is 30−40 mmHg at birth whilst in the elderly it may rise to 140−150 mmHg.

Since the cardiac output increases with exercise, so does the blood pressure, and it should be recorded only when the subject has been at rest for some time, unless a record of the pressure during exercise is required. Emotions such as fear and anxiety cause an increase in blood pressure. *Hypertension* is the name given to the condition where the blood pressure of the individual at rest is increased above normal, an increase in diastolic pressure being of greater significance than an increase in systolic pressure.

This may be due to any of the following factors.

1. Prolonged constriction of arterioles.
2. Loss of elasticity of the arterial walls.

3. An increase in viscosity of the blood, as in very severe polycythaemia.
4. Hypertension may be associated with renal disease. It is postulated that the rise in blood pressure is mediated by a hormone called renin, which is released from tissue near the glomerulae of the nephron if the glomerular blood pressure falls. Renin increases the amount of circulating angiotensin, which causes an increase in blood pressure.
5. Prolonged increase in the quantity of certain hormones which raise blood pressure, e.g. adrenaline and noradrenaline in phaeochromocytoma; serotonin in carcinoid; aldosterone in Conn's syndrome; and cortisol in Cushing's syndrome.

Hypotension (or shock) refers to a condition in which the blood pressure is lower than normal. It may be associated with:

1. Haemorrhage ⎤
2. Burns ⎬ all resulting in an actual loss of circulating fluid.
3. Severe dehydration ⎦
4. Vagal inhibition, resulting in a reduction in cardiac output.
5. Reduction in cardiac output due to sudden failure of the heart muscle.
6. Severe infective states and anaphylactic shock, where fluid is not lost from the body but is effectively lost from the circulation by stagnating in dilated vessels and/or by collecting in tissue spaces.
7. Adrenocortical insufficiency, which may increase the effects of the loss of circulating fluids in injured individuals who have been receiving corticosteroids over long periods of time.

Recording blood pressure

Principles

Blood pressure is estimated by using a sphygmo-manometer, which consists of a glass manometer containing mercury, and calibrated in millimetres. An inflatable rubber cuff, attached by a piece of tubing to the manometer, is enclosed in a cotton bag, and when applied around a limb, and inflated, acts as a tourniquet, constricting the blood vessels of the limb to which it is applied. When the pressure of the inflatable bag just exceeds the systolic blood pressure the pulsation in the artery disappears. On its return, a tapping sound can be detected by listening over the vessel wall through a stethoscope. The height of the mercury in the mano-meter at the point of the first sound gives the arterial systolic blood pressure in millimetres of mercury. As the air is let out of the bag, the sounds change in character and then disappear. Either the point at which the sounds change, or at which they disappear, may be taken as the diastolic pressure, according to the convention in the hospital. All persons recording the blood pressure of a particular patient should use the same criterion to determine the diastolic blood pressure.

Do not allow the patient to see the mercury whilst the blood pressure is being recorded, or it may cause anxiety which could increase the blood pressure.

Procedure

Ascertain whether the patient has ever had their blood pressure recorded before. If not, the semi-recumbent, relaxed position should be explained and the necessity for exposing the relevant arm from within the sleeve. The patient must be prepared for the experience of the tightness of the cuff around the upper arm at it is inflated, but assured that this will not last long and will cause no harm.

Unless otherwise stated, it is usual to record blood pressure with the patient relaxed and at rest, with the arm resting on a pillow at the side of the body, palmar surface of the hand uppermost and with the elbow flexed very slightly. The cuff of the sphygmomanometer should be placed firmly but smoothly around the arm just above the elbow, and secured, with the inflatable bag lying over the brachial artery. Both the tubing and the lower border of the cuff should be well clear of the antecubital fossa (front of the elbow). Locate the site of the brachial pulse on the ulnar side of the antecubital fossa and note its position. Palpate the radial or brachial pulse and keep the fingers lightly in position over one of these pulses whilst inflating the cuff with air. Note the height of the mercury in the manometer at the point at which the pulse disappears and continue to inflate the cuff for a further 10 to 20 mmHg. Place the stethoscope over the location of the brachial pulse (it cannot of course be felt now) and listen for the onset of the blood pressure sounds, the change in their character, and the point at which they disappear, whilst slowly deflating the sphygmomanometer cuff. Note the height of the mercury column when each of these phenomena occur. Remove the cuff from the patient's limb, leave him comfortable and chart the blood pressure. If for some reason (e.g. very low blood pressure) the blood pressure sounds cannot be heard through a stethoscope, the systolic blood pressure may be charted at the point at which the pulse can no longer be felt, although by using this method the systolic blood pressure is very slightly underestimated.

The technique of taking blood pressures should be practised on normal individuals before taking the blood pressure of ill people, since the inflated cuff can cause great discomfort.

OBSERVATION OF RESPIRATION AND RECORDING OF RESPIRATORY RATE

Respiration is the diffusion of gases between the air contained in the alveoli and the blood contained in the alveolar capillaries. The main gases involved in the exchange are oxygen, which diffuses from the alveolar air to the blood, and carbon dioxide, which diffuses from the blood to the alveolar air. The composition of the alveolar air is kept constant by the movements of respiration which ensure that the lungs alternately inflate with extra air from the environment and then deflate, expelling some of the alveolar air into the environment.

Muscles of respiration (the main ones are the intercostal muscles and the diaphragm) are voluntary muscles, but the movements of respiration are automatic. Their rhythm may be altered consciously, but not arrested deliberately over any significant period of time. However, it is important that the patient should not become self-aware whilst his respirations are being observed, or the rhythm or the rate may change.

At rest, respirations are regular, effortless and quiet, breathing out (or expiration) being merely a relaxation of the inspiratory muscles. During rest, the greater proportion of the expansion of the thoracic cavity may be due to diaphragmatic contraction rather than contraction of the intercostal muscles. At each inspiration the anterior abdominal wall moves outward slightly to allow descent of the diaphragm into the abdominal cavity. Average rates of respiration at rest are:

- Infants: 34—40/minute
- Children aged 5: about 25/minute
- Adults: 14—20/minute.

Respirations are quiet, slow and shallow in sleep, and rapid, deeper and more noisy during and after exercise, and in emotion.

Abnormalities of respiration

1. Rapid, shallow respirations may occur postoperatively if deep breathing increases the pain of an abdominal or chest wound.
2. An increase in the rate can occur in pneumonia or other infections of the respiratory tract where the volume of air entering into the lungs is restricted, or if the total alveolar surface available for gas diffusion is curtailed.
3. Increased intracranial pressure can cause either an increase in rate, the respirations assuming an automatic character, or the respirations may become very slow and shallow. Either of these phenomena should be reported, but the latter type of respiration, particularly, is a poor prognostic sign.
4. An increase in the acidity of the blood (as in diabetic coma) or in the carbon dioxide content of the blood can cause a great increase in the depth and rate of the respirations (*hyperpnoea*).
5. Respirations become noisy, or stertorous, if there is some mechanical obstruction to the passage of air in the respiratory tract. Urgent action is required to relieve the obstruction, especially if respiratory *stridor* is

present, indicating laryngeal spasm as the cause.

6. Difficulty in expiration occurs in asthmatic attacks. Respirations become noisy because of bronchiole constriction and great expiratory effort is required. Accessory muscles of respiration are used.

7. *Cheyne–Stokes* respirations occur when the respiratory centre itself is affected by lack of oxygen. The respirations become cyclical in character. A period without breathing (*apnoea*) is followed by shallow, slow respirations which increase in depth and rate to reach a crescendo, following which they get slower and shallower until apnoea occurs again.

8. Respirations become very slow and shallow when an overdosage of a depressant drug affects the respiratory centre.

Dyspnoea means difficulty in breathing. *Orthopnoea* is the term used to describe the symptom in which there is difficulty in breathing except when the individual is sitting up.

To record respiratory rate

The number of respirations is counted for half a minute and the quantity doubled to give the rate per minute. A respiration consists of both inspiration and expiration. The respirations should be counted for a full minute if there is any abnormality present of rate, rhythm or depth, or if there is any difficulty in breathing. Any of these abnormalities should, of course, be reported. For certain patients the respirations should be described in full on the initial assessment sheet (whether they are abnormal in any way or completely normal). The group of patients concerned are those with an actual or potential respiratory problem due to respiratory or heart disease, acidosis, or neurological conditions affecting respiratory muscles or respiratory centres in the brain or spinal cord. Avoid letting the patient know that the respirations are being counted.

CHARTING

A record of the temperature, pulse and respiratory rates and blood pressure is kept for each patient in the form of a graph on specially printed charts. The observation of these functions should be charted immediately, so that not only the possibility of forgetting the correct value is eliminated, but also so that the chart is always up to date. Points on the graph should be made clearly and unambiguously and joined together neatly. Observations should be made as often as necessitated by the patient's condition. It may only be necessary to record the temperature, pulse, respirations and blood pressure daily, or it may be necessary to do it as frequently as every 15 minutes. Clearly, however, the observations must be carried out with the frequency specified on the nursing care plan.

CARDIAC MONITORING

Following myocardial infarction, or cardiac surgery, continuous observation of the electrocardiogram (ECG) may be requested, so that cardiac arrhythmia may be detected the moment it occurs. This continuous observation of the ECG is made possible by its display on an oscilloscope. The electrical changes of the heart during the cardiac cycle are picked up by electrodes attached to the anterior chest wall or the limbs, and are amplified and converted into a visual picture on the screen. Nurses looking after a patient whose heart beat is being 'monitored' in this way should be capable of detecting any changes in the oscilloscope display, and of looking after the electrodes.

Electrodes may be attached to the limbs by means of straps, but more commonly they are attached to the anterior chest wall, since this gives the patient greater freedom of movement. Intimate contact between the skin and electrode is necessary to obtain a clear trace, and so all oil must be removed from the skin. The area selected is shaved, and may be on either side of the sternum, or below the nipples. It is then thoroughly cleaned by some fat solvent, such as ether, methylated spirit or acetone. Since the skin will become reddened and abraded by this thorough cleaning, the site must be changed frequently thereafter to prevent a sore. KY jelly is then spread on the electrode, which is placed on the prepared area and taped in position. It should then be connected up, and a trace displayed to ensure that it is clear, otherwise it may have to be moved. When once the trace is adequate, a loop of lead should be taped to the patient's abdomen to give freedom of movement without endangering the connection of electrode to skin.

All members of the staff should acquaint themselves with the controls on the particular oscilloscope model in use in their ward. The oscilloscope should be placed so that it can be seen easily by the nursing staff. Sometimes a second monitoring screen is placed near the nurse's station, with several channels, so that the ECGs of four or five different patients may be displayed simultaneously.

Observations which should be made

1. *Rate of heart beat.* This can be readily counted by observing the number of complete cycles traced on the screen per minute.
2. *Any change of rhythm.* In the normal ECG each trace is identical with any other trace and they occur at completely regular intervals. Any change from the ryhthm previously displayed should be reported.

Changes which should be reported

1. *Ectopic beats*. An extra, early heart beat, leaves the heart muscle refractory, so the next normal beat does not occur. The ectopic beat is then followed by a long pause and the trace is irregular.
2. *Fibrillation*. The atria contract irregularly, and the contraction may not be strong enough to trigger the ventricles into contraction. The RST complex will occur less frequently than the P waves and the whole trace will look irregular.
3. Any change in the *general condition* of the patient must be reported.

19 Fluid balance

Between 60 and 70% of the adult human body is composed of water. Since water is steadily lost from the body through evaporation, excretion, secretion, etc., it follows that a good fluid intake is essential to maintain fluid balance and thus to maintain a healthy state. For adults, a good fluid intake is 2–3 litres per day, depending on their size.

Many of the chemical substances which help to make up the composition of the body are found in solution, whilst the numerous biochemical reactions which help to maintain and develop the structure of the body and release energy also take place in solution.

Water is found both within cells and outside them. This leads to the classification of fluid as being intracellular or extracellular. Extracellular fluid is further subclassified into blood plasma and interstitial fluid. With respect to the substances which are dissolved in them, the composition of these fluids varies slightly but significantly from one another. The maintenance of the constant composition of the body fluids is crucial to life. Of particular importance in this respect are the group of substances collectively called electrolytes. Electrolytes are so-called because, in solution, molecules lose or gain one or more electrons. This renders them electrically active. Therefore they become positively or negatively charged. Individual units are called ions: the positive ones are called cations and negative ones anions. Two of the positively-charged electrolytes are of special note; these are sodium and potassium. Sodium is found in high concentrations in extracellular fluid and lower concentrations in intracellular fluid, whilst the opposite is true of potassium. This relative distribution of these cations across cell membranes is absolutely essential for normal cell function. Homeostatic action helps to maintain the balance of electrolytes. The osmotic pressure of body fluids is also crucial. (By this is meant the concentration of substances dissolved in a given quantity of liquid.) Another important variable associated with the composition of body fluids is pH. These parameters are also subject to homeostatic control, as is the total water content of the body. In particular, the kidney has an important role to play in this respect.

Homeostatic processes include:

1. The secretion of antidiuretic hormone in response to an increase of the osmotic pressure of interstitial fluid within the hypothalamus. This hormone, which is released from the pituitary gland, acts upon kidney tubules, ensuring that the minimum possible amount of water is excreted, thus conserving water.
2. The secretion of aldosterone in response to low extracellular sodium levels. This facilitates the reabsorption of sodium back into the bloodstream from the filtrate in the renal tubules. Water follows.
3. Thirst occurs as a response to increased osmotic pressure of fluid in the hypothalamus.

Clearly, the maintenance of fluid balance is complex but, equally clearly, both a normal functioning kidney and the act of drinking are important.

As mentioned above, water is lost from the body from sweating, from evaporation in expired air, from mucous membranes, and in urine and faeces. The amount lost increases if there is vomiting, diarrhoea, blood loss, burns, or seepage from wounds.

Apart from helping to maintain fluid balance by replacing fluid lost from the body, drinking liquid by mouth helps to keep the mouth moist. Moist surfaces within the mouth help us to carry out the movements essential to talking, chewing and swallowing. Moisture also ensures that we taste and smell our food, since these sensations are dependent on molecules in solution stimulating the respective sense organs.

Drinking, like eating, has become a social activity and it is customary to offer visitors a drink of some kind when they enter the home. It is important to drink sufficient fluid each day to compensate for the losses mentioned above. In hot weather or after heavy physical exercise the intake needs to be increased to compensate for sweating. The maintenance of a good level of fluid intake is particularly important for infants and elderly people. Infants have a surface area:body mass ratio larger than that of adults, which allows infants a relatively large evaporation surface. Also, a relatively high proportion of a baby's body is comprised of water, and the ratio of extracellular to intracellular water is greater. Rapid exchange between intracellular and extracellular fluids takes place. The baby's immature kidneys are unable to concentrate urine very well, leading to problems in conservation of water.

The elderly are also particularly vulnerable to the development of dehydration, but the reason is rather different. The number of active nephrons declines in age. This leads to a lower filtration rate but also to a reduced ability to reabsorb water. Frequently, elderly people have problems in getting easily to the toilet and unfortunately may reduce their fluid intake to prevent frequent micturition. This quickly leads to dehydration. Dehydration may have the effect of increasing the concentration of any drugs within the body and this increases their effects upon the person who has taken them.

Alcohol

The undesirable effects of more than a modest intake of alcohol are well known. However, alcohol has the effect of inhibiting the production of antidiuretic hormone. Therefore, following the ingestion of alcohol, the individual excretes comparatively large quantities of dilute urine. Alcohol apparently causes a depletion in intracellular fluid and this affects the brain, in particular, leading to a 'hangover'. It helps if anyone who has been drinking alcohol also drinks about a litre of water over a half-hour period.

In health, adults should aim to take in between 2 and 3 litres of liquid a day, depending upon their size. Food also provides some liquid, especially foods such as soups.

Nursing assessment of the individual's state of hydration

Clearly, from what has been said above, a person's state of hydration depends not only on water intake and loss but also on electrolyte intake and loss. Detailed accounts of the latter are beyond the scope of this book, and the remainder of this chapter will deal predominantly with fluids.

A *dehydrated* person will display some of the following characteristics:

- Thirst
- Dry, lax skin; dry mucous membranes
- Fatigue
- Reduced urine output with highly concentrated urine (providing homeostatic processes and the kidneys are functioning normally)
- Weight loss
- Sunken eyes
- Decreased venous pressure, increased temperature, pulse and respiration

A state of *overhydration* is rare, since normally the body excretes excessive liquid. However, infusion of fluids which are administered too rapidly, or kidney failure, can lead to this condition, which may be characterized by some of the following:

- Puffy eyelids
- Dependent or generalized oedema
- Ascites
- Dyspnoea
- Pleural effusion
- Increased venous pressure
- Weight gain
- Pulmonary oedema

Therefore, in assessing the patient, attention should be given to the following:

1. Any report by the patient of tiredness, fatigue or thirst.
2. The state of the patient's skin and mucous membranes.
3. Any signs of oedema.
4. Any breathlessness.

The appearance of the tissue around the eyes, temperature, pulse and respiration, and blood pressure should be recorded and any abnormality reported. Any obvious signs of increased venous pressure should be noted (swelling of the veins lying in the neck just above the clavicle, especially if this occurs in the sitting position). Aids to assessing the state of hydration include recording the weight daily (see Chapter 7). Other methods include keeping a fluid balance chart and testing urine.

FLUID BALANCE CHARTS

A fluid balance chart is a careful quantitative record of all liquid taken into the body and all liquid lost from the body (Figure 19.1). The nurse assessing a patient will decide whether or not it is necessary to keep a fluid balance record. Fluid balance charts may also be used at the request of the doctor to help in making a diagnosis or to monitor for potential or actual medical problems and the effectiveness of treatment. These charts will also be used similarly in relation to nursing problems. Some of the circumstances which suggest the need for fluid balance charts are given below.

Actual patient problems

1. If the patient is found to be dehydrated on assessment, a fluid balance chart is used to monitor the interventions used to correct dehydration and their effectiveness.
2. In oedema, output measurement is used as one means of monitoring the effectiveness of treatment. The fluid balance chart may also be used to monitor fluid intake if restriction of this has been ordered.
3. In kidney failure, the chart helps to monitor both the treatment and its effectiveness.
4. When fluid is administered intravenously, the chart will help in ensuring that the prescribed rate of administration is adhered to.
5. If there is a nasogastric tube in position, the fluid balance chart helps to ensure that dehydration is prevented from occurring due to excessive gastric suction or non-absorption. If tube feeds are being given, the chart is needed to monitor the amount of fluid being administered.
6. Whenever there is an indwelling urinary catheter in place, the chart helps in monitoring that patient has an adequate fluid intake. This helps in the prevention of urinary infection or obstruction of the catheter.
7. When a patient has diarrhoea, vomiting or excessive

INTAKE AND OUTPUT CHART

NAME *M. D. Brown*

DATE *10.1.62*   WARD *X X*   CASE No. ....

TIME	IN		OUT				NOTES
	ORAL	INTRAVENOUS	ASPIRATION	URINE	VOMIT	DRAINAGE	
1 a.m.	— — ml (cc)	*1000* ml *Dextrose/Saline* (cc)	30 ml (cc)	ml (cc)	ml (cc)	ml (cc)	*Clear fluid aspirated*
2 a.m.	*Water 30* ml	ml	24 ml	200 ml	ml	ml	"
3 a.m.	— — ml	ml	20 ml	ml	ml	ml	"
4 a.m.	— ml	ml	15 ml	ml	ml	ml	"
5 a.m.	— ml	ml	10 ml	ml	ml	ml	"
6 a.m.	*Water 30* ml	ml	20 ml	250 ml	ml	ml	"
7 a.m.	— ml	ml	36 ml	ml	ml	ml	"
8 a.m.	*Water 30* ml	ml	30 ml	ml	ml	ml	"
9 a.m.	*Water 30* ml	ml	36 ml	150 ml	ml	ml	"
10 a.m.	*Water 30* ml	*1000* ml *Dextrose 5%*	24 ml	ml	ml	ml	"
11 a.m.	*Water 30* ml	ml	16 ml	ml	ml	ml	"
12 noon	*Water 60* ml	ml	18 ml	360 ml	ml	ml	"
1 p.m.	*Water 60* ml	ml	20 ml	ml	ml	ml	"
2 p.m.	*Water 60* ml	ml	10 ml	ml	ml	ml	"
3 p.m.	*Water 60* ml	ml	24 ml	ml	ml	ml	"
4 p.m.	*Water 60* ml	ml	16 ml	500 ml	ml	ml	"
5 p.m.	*Water 60* ml	ml	18 ml	ml	ml	ml	"
6 p.m.	*Water 60* ml	ml	14 ml	ml	ml	ml	"
7 p.m.	*Water 60* ml	*1000* ml *Dextrose /Saline*	10 ml	ml	ml	ml	"
8 p.m.	*Water 60* ml	ml	10 ml	460 ml	ml	ml	"
9 p.m.	*Water 60* ml	ml	12 ml	ml	ml	ml	"
10 p.m.	— ml	ml	— ml	ml	ml	ml	
11 p.m.	— ml	ml	10 ml	ml	ml	ml	*Bile stained fluid*
12 midn't	— ml	ml	— ml	ml	ml	ml	"
24 Hour Totals	780 ml	3000 ml	432 ml	1920 ml	ml	ml	"

No.	K.	Cl.	HCO₃	Hb					
								TOTAL IN	3780 ml
								TOTAL OUT	2343 ml
135-146 mEq/1	3.8-4.6 mEq/1	98-108 mEq/1	24-28 mEq/1					BALANCE	1437 ml

Figure 19.1   Fluid balance chart.

sweating, the chart can be used to guide fluid replacement.

Potential patient problems

1. If a patient is very drowsy, monitoring the fluid intake can help to prevent dehydration.
2. Postoperatively, a fluid balance chart can help in the identification of retention of urine, oliguria or anuria.

Writing the care plan in relation to fluid balance

Instructions about nursing interventions must be clearly and concisely written, with clear goals. It is not sufficient to prescribe the fluid intake to be achieved over a 24-hour period. The amount to be achieved during each nursing shift, or even during each hour, must be specified. Patients' preferred drinks must be stated. If possible, patients should be made responsible for completing their own fluid balance charts and this will be stated on the nursing care plan. This will be the rule rather than the exception when patients are being nursed in their own homes. Clear methods of evaluation should be stated, and dates for reviewing the effectiveness of nursing intervention should be listed and adhered to.

Procedure

Fluids should be measured before they are administered to the patient and the amount he drinks should be charted straight away.

It is conventional to chart the quantity of intravenous fluid in each new container, as the unit is started or changed. If for some reason the infusion is discontinued before it has all been used, the remaining quantity should then be subtracted from the total amount. This method ensures that the chart is always up to date and is accurate, since all members of staff use the same convention.

All fluid lost from the body should be observed, measured and the quantity charted (e.g. vomit, urine). If the patient is suffering from diarrhoea, it may not be possible to measure the volume of fluid lost but an estimate should be made, so that an equivalent quantity may be replaced. It is necessary to check whether or not the patient's fluid intake and output is to be recorded before throwing away any excreta.

When accurate fluid balance measures are required, the urine collected in a urine bag must be emptied from the bag and measured in a calibrated cylinder, to prevent inaccuracies of measurement. The utensils used for measuring and collecting urine must be washed and sterilized after use to prevent cross-infection.

It was found in one research study that the volume of urine recorded using the markings on the bag overestimated the true volume of urine on 158 occasions (Jones, 1975). This was 92% of the occasions on which a check was made. On average, the degree of overestimation of urine volume using the bag markings was some 27%. This is a significant amount and could be of considerable clinical importance.

At the end of each 24-hour period the individual quantities of fluid taken in and lost from the body are added up, and attention should be drawn to any imbalance, making due allowance for fluid lost in sweating and expired air. The addition should be carried out at the same time each day, but the actual time will vary from hospital to hospital, the most common times being 24.00 hours or 08.00 hours.

NAUSEA AND VOMITING

Vomiting is a reflex action which results in the contents of the stomach being ejected through the mouth. It is usually accompanied by a feeling of nausea, and possibly faintness. Subjectively, the victim may suffer from extreme distaste and embarrassment, especially if night clothes or the bed-linen become soiled in the process.

Since nausea is usually experienced prior to vomiting, it may be possible to prevent vomiting by taking note of complaints of nausea, and reporting these to the doctor, who can then decide if an antiemetic drug is required. Care with diet and fluids, and the prevention of excessive stimulation, such as sudden movement of the patient, may also help to prevent vomiting. Deep, slow breathing accompanied by relaxation may reduce feelings of nausea. A vomit bowl and tissues should be placed within easy reach of the patient, since fear of soiling the bed may increase his anxiety level, thus increasing the likelihood of vomiting.

If the patient vomits despite all precautions, the wound should be supported by the nurse, or if there is no wound, she can support the patient's forehead. A clean vomit bowl should be provided when once the vomiting attack is over, and the patient should be given a mouth wash. Any soiled clothing must be changed, and the patient's hands and face washed if possible. The patient will probably be feeling ill, so a balance must be struck between disturbing him as little as possible and leaving him clean and comfortable.

Observations of the patient

The following should be observed.

1. Any preceding nausea or retching.
2. Whether the vomiting was associated with the intake of a particular kind of food.
3. Any regularity in the pattern of vomiting.
4. Any pain present.
5. Whether vomiting is forcible in character (projectile).

Observations of the vomit

The quantity of fluid should be measured and recorded on the fluid chart.

Appearance of vomit

The presence of certain substances in vomit can be detected by its appearance. (This method is not infallible but does give a guide.)

Poorly digested food may be seen and recognized. If the patient has been swallowing secretions from the respiratory tract, mucus may be present in the vomit. Bile, from the duodenum if present, gives vomit a brown-green colour. Frank blood can be recognized easily, whilst partially digested blood becomes dark brown in colour and unevenly distributed through the fluid due to coagulation. In intestinal obstruction, fluid which contains foul-smelling, partially digested fluid, may be vomited from the intestine. This is termed faecal vomiting. If poisoning is suspected, the vomit must be saved for analysis.

The vomit of patients with suspected or actual peptic ulceration should be tested for occult blood.

Causes of vomiting

1. *Conditions local to the gastrointestinal tract*:
   (a) Local irritation of the stomach mucosa due to drugs, irritating foods, infective states, bleeding.
   (b) Obstruction of gastrointestinal tract causing dilatation of the tract above the site of the obstruction.
2. *Excessive or unusual stimulation of peripheral nerves*:
   (a) Severe pain, especially in visceral muscles, as in renal or biliary colic.
   (b) Disturbance of the organs signalling one's position in space, as in travel sickness.

3. *Stimulation of the vomiting centre*:

(a) In severe emotion, especially if occasioned by unpleasant sights or smells.

(b) In increased intracranial pressure.

(c) If the vomiting centre is affected by disturbance of the blood chemistry, as by bacterial toxins in the bloodstream.

OBSERVATIONS OF URINE AND URINE TESTING

All urine should be measured and recorded if the patient is on a fluid chart, and even if not, the nurse should notice and report any difficulty in passing urine, any frequency, incontinence or abnormally small or large quantities being passed.

Normal urine is a clear, amber-coloured liquid, usually slightly acid in reaction and with a specific gravity of 1004 to 1030. Urine which is very dilute owing to a large fluid intake has a low specific gravity, whilst highly concentrated urine has a high specific gravity. The specific gravity of urine is the weight of a litre of the urine, compared with the weight of a litre of water. (Weight of 1 litre of pure water at 4°C = 1000 g.)

The quantity of urine passed in 24 hours depends on the fluid intake, but the average for an adult is 1500 ml. Urine consists of water, urea, uric acid, creatinine, various ions (e.g. sodium, potassium, hydrogen, chloride, ammonium and bicarbonate ions), urates, phosphates and urochrome, a pigment which gives urine its colour. An unusual appearance of urine may be due to abnormal or excessive amounts of constituents.

A sediment may settle out when urine stands and this may consist of urates or phosphates in large quantities. Urates form a pink deposit, whilst phosphates form a white one. Pus, mucus and renal tubule casts may also form a sediment when urine stands, and may render the urine cloudy. Very concentrated urine looks dark in colour. Frank bleeding may give the urine an appearance of dilute blood, whilst small amounts of blood in the urine give it a smoky, dark appearance. Urine may also appear brown or green, due to the presence of bile pigments. Thus, visual inspection may reveal the presence of some abnormalities; other abnormalities of the urine may alter its smell. Acetone in the urine gives it a sweet smell, likened to the smell of new-mown hay, whilst infection with *Escherichia coli* is associated with a fishy smell. Urine often has a smell of ammonia, which may be due to microorganisms breaking down urea to ammonia when the urine is left to stand.

Inspection of the urine may lead one to suspect that abnormalities are present, but this should always be confirmed by chemical or microbiological tests.

Simple testing of urine for the presence of abnormal constituents is carried out in the ward by nursing staff, using a specimen of urine, in the collection of which no special precautions have been taken. Such testing of urine is carried out routinely when patients are first admitted to hospital, and before general anaesthetic is administered or an operation carried out.

Ward urine testing

General principles

1. Urine should be fresh, collected in a clean, detergent-free receptacle, and carefully labelled with the patient's name.
2. All test tubes and apparatus should be clean and dry and preferably have been rinsed with distilled rather than tap water.

3. Urine should not be acidified before testing.
4. Lids should be replaced on all reagent bottles when they are not in use.
5. Reagent tablets should be handled with forceps and reagent strips should be handled only by the non-impregnated end.
6. Testing should be carried out methodically, and carefully. The results of each test should be charted immediately it has been carried out.
7. Reagent tablets and strips must be fresh. Some become unreactive if they have been exposed to the air a great deal.

Tests

1. The *appearance* of the urine is noted and recorded.
2. *Reaction*. Litmus paper is used to determine whether the urine is alkaline or acid. A drop of urine is placed on a piece of red and a piece of blue litmus paper. Acid urine turns blue litmus red, whilst alkaline urine turns red litmus blue. Urine is normally acid since the slightly alkaline reaction of the blood (pH 7.4) is maintained by adjustment made in the blood vessels surrounding the renal tubules. Excess acid or alkaline ions pass into the tubule to be excreted in the urine. The reaction of the urine varies with the diet.
3. *Specific gravity* is recorded by a urinometer, which is placed into the urine and allowed to float freely. The stem of the urinometer is calibrated, and the mark at the level at which the stem emerges from the urine gives a reading of the specific gravity; the lower level of the meniscus of the fluid should be taken. If there is insufficient urine to allow the urinometer to float free, then add an equal quantity of water, and double the final two figures of the reading obtained.

4. *Test for albumin*. Albumin is a large molecule protein found in the blood; under normal circumstances it is too large to pass through the glomerulus and into the glomerular filtrate. Occasionally it does pass into the urine in some individuals when they stand, so that urine formed in the standing position contains albumin, whilst that formed whilst the individual is lying down contains no albumin. Protein can also be found in the urine as a contaminant from vaginal secretions, or from infections of the urinary tract. However, albumin does appear in the urine in kidney damage, as in nephritis, and heart failure. Albuminuria may be an early sign of toxaemia of pregnancy.

To test for the presence of albumin in the urine, 'Albustix' reagent strips are used. The test end of the strip is dipped into the urine and removed immediately. A change of colour to green or blue-green, developing straight away, shows the presence of albumin. This colour can be compared with the chart provided to indicate the amount of albumin present.

Esbach's albuminometer can also be used to get an estimate of the quantity of albumin present. Urine should be clear, with a specific gravity of less than 1020, and acid in reaction. Thus it may be necessary to add acetic acid until it turns blue litmus pink; filter, or dilute the urine with a known quantity of distilled water. The tube of the albuminometer should be filled to mark U with urine, and to mark R with Esbach's reagent. It is then corked, mixed by inversion several times, and left undisturbed for 24 hours, after which time the height of the precipitate which forms at the bottom of the tube is read off on the graduated scale indicating grams of protein per 100 g of urine.

5. *Test for glucose*. Glucose appears in the urine when the blood level of glucose exceeds the renal threshold

for glucose, i.e. approximately 180 mg per 100 ml. The renal threshold for glucose may be exceeded in normal individuals immediately after meals with a heavy carbohydrate content, if their renal threshold is on the lower side of normal. Glucose also appears in the urine of individuals suffering from diabetes mellitus, whose blood sugar level rises and remains high for a considerable time after a meal. Small amounts appear in the urine in pituitary and thyroid disease, head injury and subarachnoid haemmorhage.

Glycosuria can be detected by the use of 'Clinistix' reagent strips. The test end of one of these should be dipped into the specimen of urine and then removed. A positive result, indicating the presence of glucose, is shown by a blue colour developing at the moistened end of the strip within 10 seconds.

A quantitative estimation of the glucose present can be obtained by using 'Clinitest' reagent tablets. These tablets must be fresh for accurate results. Five drops of urine are placed into a clean test-tube, using a pipette. The pipette should be rinsed with distilled water, and then 10 drops of water added to the urine, followed by the Clinitest tablet. The latter will cause agitation of the solution. Fifteen seconds after the agitation has ceased, the test-tube should be shaken gently and the resultant colour matched with one of the colours on the chart provided to indicate the quantity of glucose in the specimen. Whilst 'Clinistix' react only with glucose, 'Clinitest' tablets react with other sugars, such as lactose (which may be present in the urine of pregnant women), galactose and fructose, and other reducing substances such as ascorbic acid and salicylate metabolites.

6. *Test for ketones* (acetone and acetoacetate). Ketones

accumulate in the bloodstream when excess quantities of fat are being metabolized in the absence of the metabolism of adequate quantities of glucose. This may occur in diabetes mellitus and in starvation, in both of which conditions acetone and acetoacetate will be excreted in the urine as the blood level increases. The presence of ketone in the urine of a diabetic patient should be reported, since diabetic coma occurs as a result of large quantities of ketone bodies in the bloodstream and not as a result of the high blood glucose.

'Acetest' reagent tablets are used to test urine for the presence of acetone and acetoacetate. One tablet is placed on a clean surface, such as a white tile or piece of paper, and one drop of urine is added. A colour change at the end of 30 seconds exactly should be matched with the scale provided, a positive result being shown by a pale lavender to a strong mauve colour.

'Ketostix' reagent strips also react with acetone and acetoacetate. The test end of the strip should be dipped into a fresh specimen of urine, and removed immediately. Excess moisture should be removed by touching the strip briefly on the side of the container. Fifteen seconds later, the colour should be compared with the chart provided. The presence of acetoacetate or acetone is indicated by a lavender or purple colour.

7. *Test for the presence of blood in urine.* Large quantities of blood in the urine will be obvious to the naked eye, but it may be necessary to test for the presence of blood in the urine, which may be present in small quantities in infective lesions and nephritis.

'Hemastix' reagent strips react to haemoglobin. The test end should be dipped into the urine and removed immediately. Thirty seconds later the test end should be matched with the colour chart. A positive result is shown by the development of a blue colour.

8. *Test for bilirubin*. Bilirubin is a product of the metabolism of haemoglobin. It is conjugated in the liver, and in this form it can pass through the glomerulus into the glomerular filtrate. Since it is normally secreted from the liver in the bile, it does not appear in the urine in this form, but in the form of urobilin and urobilinogen which are formed from the further breakdown of conjugated bilirubin. The blood concentration of conjugated bilirubin rises if the flow of bile is obstructed in any way, and bilirubin appears in the urine.

'Ictotest' reagent tablets are used to test for bilirubin in urine. Five drops of urine should be placed on a special test mat, and the reagent tablets placed in the middle of the moist area. Two drops of urine are then flowed over the tablet. The colour of the test mat *around* the tablet should be observed 30 seconds later. A positive result is indicated by a blush-purple colour on the paper around the tablet.

OBSERVATION OF SPUTUM

Excessive secretions from the respiratory tract are coughed up, a process called expectoration, the expectorated secretions being called sputum. A patient should be discouraged from swallowing sputum, and a disposable sputum carton should be provided, together with tissues to wipe the mouth. The quantity and type of sputum should be noted, and the ease with which it is coughed up. If there should be any difficulty in expectoration, then physiotherapy, inhalations or expectorants may be ordered by the doctor to help liquefy the sputum.

Sputum may be predominantly *mucoid* in character, as

in the early stages of inflammatory conditions such as pneumonia or bronchitis. *Mucopurulent* sputum may be coughed up in bronchiectasis, or if a lung abscess ruptures. The sputum may be *blood-stained* in pneumonia, in pulmonary infarction, tuberculosis, and carcinoma of the bronchus. If a large amount of blood is present, it may be bright red and frothy. The coughing up of fresh blood is termed *haemoptysis*. Sputum may be very *frothy* when the pulmonary blood pressure is raised, giving pulmonary oedema.

OBSERVATION OF RATES OF INFUSION

Infusion tubing incorporating a special 'drip chamber' allows fluids to be administered slowly over long periods of time at a constant rate of drips. Infusions may be used to administer fluids into the following tissues or areas: (1) intravenous, (2) subcutaneous, (3) intragastric, or (4) rectal.

Since there is a greater risk of complications from intravenous infusion than any of the others, the observations required whilst an intravenous infusion is in progress will be described. If blood is administered by this means, then it is termed a blood transfusion.

Observation of the patient having a blood transfusion

1. Careful checking is needed to ensure that the bottle of blood being transfused is the bottle of donor blood which has been cross-matched with the patient's blood and found to be compatible with it.
2. The patient's temperature, pulse and respiration rates should be recorded at frequent intervals, and a fluid intake and output chart kept. A mild incompatibility reaction may be reflected in a rise of a temperature.

3. Empty blood bottles should be returned to the laboratory unwashed.

Observation of the patient whilst an intravenous infusion or transfusion is in progress

1. Frequent observation of the rate of administration is needed. This should be regulated, if necessary, to match the prescribed rate in terms of drops per minute.
2. Inspection of the site of the insertion of the needle or catheter should be made to ensure that it is securely within the vein and that no fluid is leaking subcutaneously. Some intravenous fluids can cause damage if allowed to get into subcutaneous tissue, e.g. blood, noradrenaline, urea.
3. The level of fluid within the bottle or infusion container must be watched to ensure that it never completely empties, otherwise air will get into the tubing and this is very difficult to remove. An exchange should be made for a full container whilst there is still a very small amount of fluid left in the old one. Tubing must be clipped off whilst the bottle is changed, and sterility must be preserved.
4. Care must be taken that the fluid given is that which has been prescribed.
5. The infusion may stop completely. Among the reasons why this could happen are the following:
   (a) Accidental clipping off of the tubing.
   (b) Blood clot blocking the needle or catheter.
   (c) Occlusion of the needle because it is displaced in the vein and its lumen is resting against the vein wall.
   (d) Spasm, or compression of the vein above the infusion. In general, the nurse deals with factors affecting the tubing, whilst the doctor deals with factors involving adjustment of the needle within the vein.

6. When once the infusion has been discontinued, the vein site should be observed for signs of inflammation.

WOUND DISCHARGES AND DRAINS

Bleeding immediately postoperatively may stain the dressings of the wound, which should be repacked. A drain may have been inserted into the wound at operation to allow for the drainage of any anticipated collection of fluid which could delay healing. The drain is often shortened before it is removed, and observation of the type and amount of discharge should be made whenever the wound is dressed. Discharge will usually consist of stale blood unless the wound becomes infected, in which case it may be purulent.

Occasionally, some kind of suction is needed to help the drainage of discharge from a wound. This may be provided by apparatus such as a Roberts' low pressure pump or by some form of vacuum drainage such as a Redivac bottle. Whatever apparatus is used, the amount of drainage should be measured, sterility being ensured whilst the apparatus is changed.

Special types of drains may be inserted into deep tissues. Following an operation on the common bile duct, a T-tube may be inserted with the short arms of the 'T' lying within the lumen of the common bile duct and the long arm emerging from the wound, and draining into a sterile, closed container at the side of the bed. The quantity of bile should be measured carefully and the tubing replaced into a fresh sterile container; the colour of the drainage should also be noted. This T-tube is removed by the medical officer when drainage stops, and an X-ray, with the use of a radio-opaque contrast medium, shows the common bile duct to be functional. The use of an analgesic is needed before removal of the tube.

PART IV: Some therapeutic techniques

20 Dressing technique

Dressings are carried out for the following reasons:

1. To remove soiled dressings (which may encourage the multiplication of microorganisms) and to replace them with clean, sterile dressings.
2. To place a protective cover over a broken area of skin.
3. To remove stitches or clips; to shorten or remove drainage tubes.

Dressing a wound is a potential source of cross-infection, since, by definition, a wound is an interruption in the continuity of the protective surface of the body (skin). Microorganisms can thereby gain direct access to the body, which provides ideal conditions for their growth. An understanding of microbiology and a scrupulous technique are needed if infection is to be avoided. Infection delays wound healing, at the very least, and may even cause the death of the patient at the worst.

General principles involved in performing dressings

1. Since there is a danger from airborne organisms in carrying out a dressing, however good the technique, dressings should never be carried out unnecessarily. An operation wound which has been sutured or clipped with no drain inserted should heal well, with no complications. Such a wound need be dressed only when the sutures and clips are to be removed.

2. All instruments and dressings which will come into contact with the wound must be sterile.

3. Since the wound will be uncovered during the procedure, the number of microorganisms in the air and the disturbance of the air should be reduced to a minimum. At least 1 hour should have lapsed after ward cleaning, bed-making or furniture-moving activities, before dressings are carried out. If possible, the dressing should be carried out in a room specially designated for the purpose.

4. The technique should be such that the wound is exposed for the minimum time possible.

5. Movement of staff within the ward, movement of staff and visitors in and out of the ward, and movement of relatives in the home setting, must be curtailed whilst dressings are carried out, unless there is a special clinic room in which dressings can be done.

6. Unused dressings should be placed for autoclaving and must not be carried from the bed to bed.

7. Anything which is taken from bed to bed (e.g. the trolley, the lotion bottle) should be washed over with antiseptic lotion and thoroughly dried between each dressing, so that possible contamination is reduced to a minimum.

8. Any wound known to be infected should be dressed last of all if a series of dressings is being carried out.

Basic dressing trolley

Requirements

The trolley should be made of light, washable material, and it should be smooth running and quiet in use. It should be thoroughly washed before starting the dressings and after each dressing, with an antiseptic detergent solution (e.g. Savlon). If possible, this solution should be sprayed on, then the trolley should be dried thoroughly with clean, absorbent, paper towels.

An alternative method is to wash the trolley thoroughly with soap and water and to dry it. Then a prepacked sterile swab soaked in spirit can be used to wipe the trolley immediately before use.

Top shelf

A sterile pack which contains sufficient material to carry out the dressing is placed on the top shelf of the trolley. A basic dressing pack will contain wool balls, gauze swabs and sterile towels (Figure 20.1). A gallipot and four pairs of forceps (Spencer Wells, dissecting or dressing forceps can be used) may be included, or supplied in separate packs. Larger packs may include more dressings and a roll of cotton wool. Other instruments which may be required, such as stitch scissors, clip removers, safety pin, large bandage scissors, may be included in the appropriate pack, or may be supplied in individual containers.

Bottom shelf

A bottle of lotion, if prescribed for the dressing, will be taken to the bedside. The outside of the bottle should be washed with antiseptic solution and dried, as described for the trolley above.

Sufficient adhesive tape, bandage, tubular gauze, elastic net etc. to fix the dressing in place should be placed on the trolley.

A disposal bag for dirty dressings and a container for dirty instruments will be required.

Note. If the dressings are sterilized and stored in a bag, this may be used as a container for the dirty dressings once the pack has been opened.

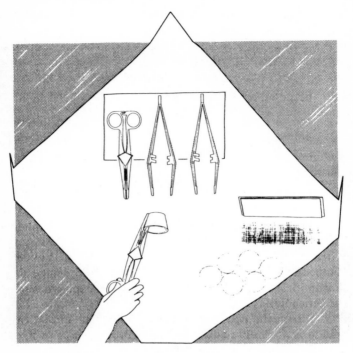

Figure 20.1 Basic dressing pack opened out. Equipment arranged using handling forceps.

Masks

Masks are commonly worn to filter microorganisms from the expired air, both during the preparation of the trolley, and to carry out the dressing. These masks may be made of paper or gauze. Cellophane paper may be inserted into the gauze masks to provide a more adequate filter of the expired air.

Certain precautions are necessary when wearing a mask

to prevent it from being a positive danger to the patient, rather than a safeguard.

A paper mask should be worn only for a maximum of 15 minutes at a time or it will become so dampened from the water vapour content of the expired air that it is no longer efficient.

The mask must be adjusted correctly, so that it covers the nostrils and the mouth.

Care is needed in removing the mask. It should be handled by the tapes or elastic, and the body of the mask should not be touched. The mask should be placed directly into the pedal-action bin provided for it, and the hands washed straight away.

Basic dressing procedure

Two nurses should carry out this procedure, one to do the dressing (dresser) and one as assistant (assistant).

1. Prepare the trolley, making sure that everything which will be needed is on it.
2. Take the trolley to the patient's bedside, and explain the procedure to the patient, in terms he will understand. Alternatively, the patient may be taken to the dressing room. In this case, he will need to have had explained the reason for moving, as well as having an explanation of the procedure.
3. Explanations given to the patient should include the following information:
   (a) What is to be done and why,
   (b) How long it will take.
   (c) What it will feel like, e.g. explain the coldness of any lotion, any pulling when an old dressing is removed or when stitches or clips are removed.
   (d) What the patient can do to help to make the procedure less uncomfortable, by relaxation or

deep breathing, for example, or position; also, if the patient can help the nurse in any way.

(e) That information will be given throughout the procedure.

4. Screen the bed and position the patient so that the wound is accessible and he is as comfortable as possible. Then turn back the bedclothes and place a flannelette sheet or bedjacket over the patient to keep him warm.

5. The nurse who is to carry out the dressing should wash and dry the hands thoroughly.

6. The assistant then opens the dressing pack. If the dressings are contained in a bag, they are slid gently within the towel wrapping from the bag, on to the trolley, and the bag is placed either on the bottom shelf or attached to the side rail with the adhesive tape from the pack, so that it can be used as a disposal bag.

7. Whether there is an outer bag or not, the towel wrapping the dressings should be carefully opened by the dresser, and spread out on the top shelf, touching the outer surface only. This forms a sterile working surface on the trolley, when once it is spread, so that the previously outer surface is in contact with the trolley surface and the inner surface is facing upwards and has been kept sterile. Next, a pair of forceps should be picked up. If they are in a separate container, the assistant can open this, whilst the dresser extracts them very carefully, touching only the handle. If they are in the main pack, the dresser picks them up by the handle, ensuring that the pack contents are not contaminated in the process. She can then use these forceps to arrange the pack contents on the sterile surface as desired. It is a good idea to have a well-defined surface on which the forceps can be

rested if needed again. This can be a gauze swab, or better still, a kidney dish.

8. The assistant now pours any lotion, and opens the packs containing extra instruments which are needed. Great care must be taken that the assistant touches only the outside of the pack. The dresser can take the contents and place them on the sterile working surface, using the first pair of forceps.

9. Now the assistant removes any bandages, or loosens the adhesive tape, holding the dressing in position, so the dressing can be removed by the dresser, using two pairs of forceps, which are then discarded.

10. Two fresh pairs of forceps are used to arrange a sterile towel over the skin near the wound, and then the dressing is carried out.

Principles of dressing a wound

1. Antiseptics should not be used unless it is absolutely necessary. Antiseptic lotions may damage healthy skin and disrupt the migration of cells involved in the healing process.

2. If lotion is used, wring the swab out with the forceps to remove as much moisture as possible. Swab from the wound out. Never swab in toward the wound, since this sweeps microorganisms which are harmless on the intact skin into the wound, where they can do harm.

3. Dry the area, using cotton wool swabs.

4. If dressings are to be placed over the wound, place them so that they completely cover and protect the wound. If strapping is used to hold the dressings in position, it should be applied so that the patient can move freely without dislodging a corner of the dressing. Keep the patient informed throughout the procedure.

Whenever a dressing is being performed, it should be carried out as gently as possible. The patient's facial and vocal expressions can be noted to ensure that he is not being hurt unnecessarily, since it is more difficult to estimate the exact amount of pressure to be exerted using forceps than when a procedure is carried out using one's fingers or hands.

When the dressing has been completed, any old plaster marks can be removed, and the patient is repositioned by the assistant whilst the dresser takes the trolley, disposes of all the used articles, and cleans it thoroughly, ready for the next dressing.

Removal of stitches

The exact technique for removing stitches depends upon the way in which they have been inserted.

1. Cut the stitch so that, in withdrawing it, no part of the stitch which was exposed to the air is dragged through the tissues.
2. Ensure that the cut is made in such a way that no piece of stitch is left in the tissues.
3. It is easier, if all the sutures to be removed are cut, holding the stitch scissors or stitch cutter (Figure 20.2) in the right hand, and a pair of dissecting forceps in the left hand, to lift the knot of the stitch so the stitch can be cut between the knot and the skin.
4. The scissors or stitch cutter can then be discarded and a second pair of dressing or dissecting forceps are taken into the right hand for removing the stitch from the skin. Gently lay the dressing forceps, held in the left hand, over the skin area, in the same plane as the skin to prevent the skin from being pulled when the stitch is withdrawn.

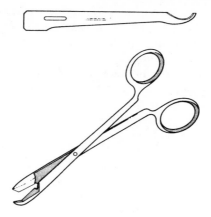

Figure 20.2 Stitch cutter and clip removers.

5. Commonly, half the stitches (alternate ones) are removed on one day, and the rest the following day.

Removal of clips

Special clip-removing forceps are used for the removal of
clips. Take the clip removers in the right hand and a pair
of dissecting or dressing forceps in the left hand. Steadying
the clip with the dressing forceps, insert one blade of the
clip removers under the centre of the clip, and one blade
over the centre of the clip. Ensure the blades are inserted
for a sufficient distance. Gently squeeze the blades
together. This straightens the clip metal, lifting it from
the skin on either side.

To shorten a drain

The procedure for shortening a drain is as follows.

1. Using forceps, open the sterile safety pin and place it on the sterile area, ready for use.
2. Clean the area around the drain, using wool swabs and lotion as necessary.
3. Remove any stitch holding the drain in position.
4. Gently turn the drain within the wound, to loosen it, if it is a tubular drain.
5. Grasp the protruding end of the drain with a pair of artery forceps and clip them into position.
6. Using these forceps, gently ease the drain out of the wound for the prescribed distance, e.g. 13–25 mm.
7. Take another pair of artery forceps and pick up the sterile safety pin. Grasping the pin firmly in the forceps, pass it through the tube, and out the other side, as near to the skin surface as possible. Great care is needed not to injure the patient; the pin should be directed in a slightly upward direction away from the skin. The second pair of forceps can be used to steady the tubing. Close the pin, using two pairs of forceps.
8. Cut excess tubing off, using sterile bandage scissors.

Removal of a drain

The method of removing a drain is as above, except that the drain is removed completely at step (6).

Note. A different technique is required for the removal of a water-seal drain or T-tube. These are usually removed by a medical officer.

Dressing technique when there is only one nurse available

If one individual has to carry out a dressing by herself, it is far more difficult to achieve an aseptic technique. The nurse should have a good knowledge of microbiology, and carry out the dressing as conscientiously as possible.

The trolley is prepared as previously described, and

taken to the bedside. Explanation is given to the patient, the bed is screened, and the patient positioned. The bedclothes are turned back and the patient is kept warm with a flannelette blanket.

Next, the dressing is loosened, but left in position to protect the wound. The nurse washes her hands, and then opens the pack as described previously, arranging the contents on the sterile surface with a pair of forceps. Any extra forceps or equipment required must be taken out of the packs and arranged on the sterile area. If lotion is required, it should be poured out. Using a second pair of forceps if necessary, the dressing is removed from the wound into the disposal bag, and the forceps discarded. Using fresh forceps, the wound is dressed as described above.

Dressing wounds in the patient's own home

The principles of carrying out dressings are the same, whether in hospital or in the patient's own home. However, the materials used for the dressing by the community nurse are bought on prescription and so are the property of the patient. Improvisation may be required in relation to equipment, and clearly there is no dressing trolley available on which to set out the equipment. Instead, a clean space is used on a convenient table, tray or the patient's bed. The nurse may need to go to the bathroom or kitchen for handwashing as there is unlikely to be a washbasin in the sitting room or bedroom.

It may be difficult to maintain absolute sterility throughout the whole of the procedure. However, micro-organisms which may contaminate instruments or dressing materials are mainly those from the patient and/or relatives and are unlikely to be pathogenic to the patient. They are extremely unlikely to be antibiotic-resistant.

21 Administration of drugs

Drugs are substances obtained from vegetable, mineral and animal sources and used for medicinal purposes. They may be introduced into the body in various forms and by various routes. Drugs may be dispensed in liquid form, as solutions, tinctures, infusions, emulsions or oils, or in solid form, as pills, powders, tablets or capsules.

Drugs may be administered by mouth, occasionally by the rectum, or parenterally, that is to say they may be introduced by routes other than the alimentary tract, such as subcutaneous, intramuscular or intravenous injections, or by inhalation.

Within the hospital, medicines for administration by mouth must be stored in a cupboard reserved for this purpose, and substances intended for external application only must be kept in a separate cupboard.

Drugs controlled by the Misuse of Drugs Act (1971)

The Misuse of Drugs Act (1971) controls the sale and use of substances liable to cause drug addition. Opium and its alkaloids, notably morphine, cocaine and Indian hemp, were the drugs controlled by the original Act; more recent additions are pethidine hydrochloride and methadone hydrochloride (Physeptone). These drugs may be supplied to the public only on the written prescription of a medical practitioner. Hospital wards and departments are, however, authorized to keep a stock of certain preparations, such as morphine and pethidine, but they must be ordered on a duplicate form signed by the authorized responsible person, i.e. the sister or charge nurse who is responsible for the safe storage of the drugs and for ensuring that they are used only in accordance with written orders of the medical staff. Controlled drugs must be kept in a locked cupboard reserved for the storage of these drugs, the key of which is kept by a registered nurse or a state enrolled nurse who has received additional training in relation to drugs; the containers are supplied to the ward in a locked box. All prescriptions and order forms must be kept by the hospital for a period of 2 years from the date of issue.

Scheduled poisons

The Poisons and Pharmacy Act controls the sale, prescription and use of a very large range of substances which are potentially toxic or dangerous. There are schedules under the Act which list a great number of poisonous substances and the regulations to be observed in their use. Some of these are of particular importance in medical and nursing practice.

The schedules list drugs which are to be used only on prescription and under medical supervision. Within hospital practice these drugs can be obtained from the pharmacist's department only on the written order of a medical officer or the sister or charge nurse of the ward or department. They must be clearly labelled as poisons and stored in a locked cupboard, the key of which must be kept on the person of a registered nurse or specially trained enrolled nurse. These drugs should be checked regularly by the nurse in charge of the ward, but a ward record book is not necessary.

Scheduled poisons are usually obtained from the phar-

macy by using a special order book. Each order should
be signed by sister, charge nurse or deputy.

The Therapeutic Substances (Prevention of Misuse) Act

A number of other drugs are potentially dangerous and
are controlled by further legislation. In practice these are
treated with the same precautions as scheduled poisons.
These include insulin, corticosteroids for systemic use,
hypotensive agents, paraldehyde and anticoagulants. The
last should be stored in a locked refrigerator.

Drugs and community nursing practice

A major difference between community nursing practice
and hospital nursing practice is the fact that the drugs
used in treatment are the property of patients within the
community. In contrast, in hospital, drugs prescribed by the
hospital doctors belong to the hospital, although obviously
any drugs which the patients bring from home when they
are admitted to hospital continue to belong to the patients.

The community nurse will clearly be aware of those
drugs which have been prescribed for any patients in the
caseload. It is part of the role of the community nurses to
advise patients, relatives, and/or other informal carers
about the safe use and storage of drugs. The latter is
particularly important if there are children in the household. Optimum conditions for storing drugs, accuracy in
relation to the time of taking drugs, potential side-effects,
and safe disposal of any remaining drugs at the end of
treatment are all issues on which the family will need
advice.

Drugs which are subject to the Misuse of Drugs Act
will be prescribed by the general practitioner. The nurse
will be aware of these and will maintain a record of the
number of doses issued, the number used and the number

of doses remaining. This record may well be held at the health centre from which the nurse works.

ADMINISTRATION OF DRUGS BY MOUTH

Drugs must be given punctually. In hospital practice, the standard times for giving 4-hourly, 6-hourly drugs, and those given twice, or three times a day, should be known, and the times adhered to by all members of staff. In this way errors can be avoided. It is important for many drugs that the blood concentration is not allowed to fall below a given level, so an interval longer than that prescribed must not be allowed to lapse. For other drugs, two doses given closer together than prescribed might increase the blood concentration to a dangerous level.

Method of pouring medicine

The method of pouring medicine is as follows.

1. Shake the bottle.
2. Hold the bottle with the label uppermost to prevent soiling of the label. (**Note**. A bottle with a label which does become soiled, or illegible for any other reason at all, must be returned to the pharmacy.)
3. Remove the cork, holding it in the little finger of the left hand.
4. Measure the dose into the medicine glass, holding the glass at eye level.
5. If there is a sediment, provide a glass rod to stir the medicine, immediately before the patient takes it.

Pills, tablets, capsules or *cachets* should be placed into a special disposable container, a spoon, or a medicine glass, before being taken to the patient.

Procedure for administration of medicines and other oral drugs

The procedure for administration of medicine and other oral drugs is given as follows.

1. Collect the patient's prescription sheets and a container for the drug, and check that the dose has not already been given.
2. Select the correct drug from the cupboard or drug trolley. Check the name of the drug and strength supplied against the prescription sheet. **Note.** Although a nurse is never responsible for prescribing drugs, it is important that she knows the uses, action, side-effects, and usual dose of any drug which she administers to a patient. Such knowledge helps a nurse to recognize any discrepancy between the normal dose and the prescribed dose of a drug. If there is such a discrepancy, she should check with the doctor that the name and dose of the drug written on the prescription sheet are as he intended before administering the drug.
3. Measure the correct dose.
4. Take the dose to the bedside with the prescription sheet.
5. Check the patient's name, the drug and the dose against the prescription sheet.
6. Give the drug to the patient. Ensure that he swallows it, with some water if necessary.
7. Record that the drug has been given if it is an antibiotic, night sedation or a drug prescribed *p.r.n.* (*pro re nata*).

Note. If the drug is a scheduled poison, the whole procedure must be checked by a second person, who must witness that the correct drug is given to the right patient. In practice, however, most hospitals insist that all drug administration is checked by two members of the nursing staff.

The prescription sheet referred to above must be the one on which the order signed by the doctor is written.

Administration of a dangerous drug

Two persons must witness the collection of the correct dose of a dangerous drug and its administration; one of these should be a registered nurse or a medical practitioner.

1. Collect the prescription sheet with the written order signed by the doctor, and the ward record book.
2. Check that the patient has not been given the drug.
3. Select the correct drug from the controlled drug cupboard.
4. Find the entry for this drug in the ward record book and check the total quantity of the drug against the quantity which has been previously administered.
5. Check the dose into a container or syringe and lock up the unused ampoules or tablets.
6. Enter the patient's name, the dose of the drug and the date in the record book.
7. Take the drug and the prescription sheet to the bedside, and check the patient's name, the name and dose of the drug against the prescription. Make quite certain the dose has not been given already.
8. Give the drug.
9. Enter the time of administration and the signatures of the two nurses into the record book. Record the administration of the dose into the Kardex and on the prescription sheet.

General remarks

Many medicines have an unpleasant taste, and the majority of patients can be allowed a drink of water, a piece of fruit or a sweet to take away the taste.

Holding the nose while drinking is sometimes a help, as taste depends to some extent on smell.

A medicine containing iron stains the teeth and should be taken through a glass drinking tube or a straw. The mouth should be washed out afterwards and the teeth cleaned.

Powders are most easily swallowed if put upon the tongue and washed down with a drink of water.

Pills and capsules are swallowed with a drink of water. Some pills (e.g. prednisone, phenylbutazone, aspirin) are acid and can cause stomach upset if given when the stomach is empty. It is helpful to give a glass of milk with the pills. Some of this can be taken before the pills and the rest may be used to help swallow the pills.

Antibiotics should be given when the stomach is empty.

Oily substances are difficult to take, not only on account of the flavour, but also because of the disagreeable taste of oil in the mouth. For an adult patient the oil must be prepared so that the patient can drink it all at once without tasting it. One method is to warm a china measure or medicine glass in hot water; about 2 teaspoonfuls (10 ml) of lemon or mixed lemon and orange juice are poured into the measure and the prescribed dose of the oil floated on top of this. More fruit juice is poured on to the top of the oil. A slice of lemon or orange may be taken to the bedside with the dose. The patient is told to bite the piece of lemon, then swallow the dose at one gulp and bite the slice of lemon again.

The disadvantages of giving drugs by mouth are:

1. The patient may not be able or may refuse to swallow the dose.
2. The drug may be only partially absorbed.
3. The drug may irritate the alimentary tract, causing

vomiting or acting as a purgative, so that the desired effect is lost.

ADMINISTRATION OF DRUGS BY THE RECTUM

Drugs may be administered per rectum, either in the form of suppositories (e.g. aminophylline) or as solutions. The method is the same as for the administration of other types of suppository or retention enema (see Chapters 9 and 23).

GIVING DRUGS BY INHALATION

Drugs given by inhalation may be used for their general effect or for their local action on the respiratory tract. The drug must be in the form of a vapour or a liquid which readily vaporizes, or a fine spray, such as an aerosol spray. Anaesthetic gases are examples of drugs exerting a general effect when inhaled. Aromatic substances, such as menthol and tincture of benzoin, may be added to steam inhalations for their local effect in the treatment of upper respiratory tract infections, such as acute sinusitis and laryngitis (see Chapter 13). An aerosol spray of an antispasmodic drug may be ordered in the treatment of asthma.

LATIN WORDS AND ABBREVIATIONS USED IN PRESCRIPTION WRITING

Latin and its abbreviations are falling into disuse because of the ease with which terms can be misread. Nurses should seek clarification of any term used on the prescription sheet which is not understood.

22 Parenteral administration of drugs

Drugs may be given by injection when rapid action is required, if the drug is destroyed by intestinal secretions, if it is not absorbed from the alimentary tract or if the patient is unable to take the drug orally for some reason.

As mentioned in the previous chapter, in community nursing practice, drugs remain the property of the patient, and this applies equally to drugs administered by injection. There are some categories of drug which the patients may learn to inject for themselves in their own home. Insulin is an obvious example. The new pen-type devices for administration of insulin aid self-injection. There is no reason why patients and/or relatives should not learn to administer other drugs by hypodermic injection, but this is not common practice, except in the case of insulin.

Occasionally, for patients who are suffering severe pain drugs may be administered by means of an electronic pump, either subcutaneously or intravenously. This pump is usually under the patient's own control. He or she will have been taught how to use this by a doctor or clinical nurse specialist.

Other types of injections which may be required less frequently are usually administered by the community nurse. An example, is Cytamin (vitamin B_{12}) for patients with anaemia. This is a drug which is administered by intramuscular injection.

In hospital practice, whenever a drug is given to a

patient by injection the dose should be checked and the whole procedure observed by a second nurse.

HYPODERMIC INJECTION

Hypodermic (or subcutaneous) injection is the method commonly used when only a small volume of fluid is to be injected and when the solution is not likely to damage the superficial tissues. Drugs which may be irritant in the subcutaneous tissue must be injected either into muscle, which has a good blood supply, or into a vein. It should also be noted that, if the superficial circulation is depleted, absorption of a substance injected hypodermically is likely to be slow and uncertain. Therefore morphine, for example, should be given intravenously to a patient suffering from severe shock.

Drugs for hypodermic injection are usually dispensed in solution, either in single dose ampoules, which provide a considerable safeguard against accidental overdosage, or in multidose containers. Tablets which are dissolved in sterile water immediately before use are also obtainable and, although not often seen in hospitals now, they may be used in private practice. The usual sites for injection are the outer aspect of the upper arm or the thigh.

Syringes of 1 or 2 ml capacity are used, with size 17 to 20 needles. Disposable needles and syringes, used for one injection only, are supplied in hospital.

The syringe in its container should be placed on a tray, together with a spray bottle of skin-cleansing antiseptic and sterile wool swabs.

The tray with the drug, and the patient's prescription sheet, should be taken to a second person to be checked. If the drug is one covered by the Dangerous Drugs Act, the book should also be taken to the second person who should be a registered nurse.

Solutions for hypodermic injections may be dispensed in multidose rubber-capped bottles. The bottle should be held so that the cap is not handled. After wiping the cap of the bottle with a swab moistened with alcohol, the needle should be pushed through the centre of the cap and a little air injected to facilitate the removal of the fluid. Slightly more than the required quantity of the solution should be taken up, and then, holding the syringe with the needle vertical, the piston is pushed up until the edge is on a level with the line showing the required number of millitres.

If the drug is in a glass ampoule, a file may be required to make a mark on the neck of the ampoule where it is to be broken. The outside of the glass is washed with a swab, moistened with alcohol and, holding the ampoule in a piece of sterile gauze to prevent splintered glass from cutting the nurse, the neck is then broken at the file mark or at the spot marked by the manufacturer.

If the patient is not familiar with the procedure, the nurse should explain what she is about to do and that a small scratch will be felt. An injection made with a sharp needle is scarcely felt, although the patient will feel pressure within the subcutaneous tissue as the liquid is injected, and should be warned of this.

The site of the injection may be rubbed fairly vigorously with a swab moistened with alcohol, in order both to cleanse the skin and to increase the blood supply. A small piece of skin and subcutaneous tissue should be taken up between the thumb and first finger of the left hand, pulling the skin fairly taut. The needle is inserted quickly and firmly into the fold of subcutaneous tissue at an angle of 45° and the piston pushed steadily down. The swab should be pressed on the skin while the needle is withdrawn.

Great care should be taken with needles after use. As

mentioned in Chapter 5, they must not be resheathed and must be disposed of safely in the special bin provided. Any accidental needle stick injury suffered by the nurse must be formally reported in writing.

Among the drugs commonly given by hypodermic injection are adrenaline and insulin.

INTRAMUSCULAR INJECTION

Drugs may be given intramuscularly when larger amounts are to be injected than can be given by hypodermic injection, when more rapid action is needed, and this method is also chosen when the drug would be irritating if injected superficially. The sites usually chosen are the vastus externus muscle of the outer aspect of the thigh, the gluteal muscles of the buttock, or the deltoid muscle in the upper part of the arm (Figure 22.1). It is essential to avoid giving the injection into a blood vessel, nerve or periosteum. To ascertain that the needle is not in a vein, the plunger should be withdrawn a little; if blood is drawn up into the syringe, then a vein has been punctured and the needle must be withdrawn, reinjected and the plunger once more withdrawn before giving the injection. When making an injection into the buttock, the upper and outer quadrant should be chosen, as there is a risk of stabbing the sciatic nerve if the needle is inserted too near the sacrum. The periosteum can be avoided by giving the injection into a site where there is plenty of muscle covering the bone and by not stabbing too deeply.

The injection and the skin over the site are prepared in the manner described for the giving of hypodermic injections. The size of syringe and needles required will depend on the amount and type of the drug to be injected and on the site of the injection, 1-, 2- or 5-ml syringes may be needed, and needles 5–6 cm long.

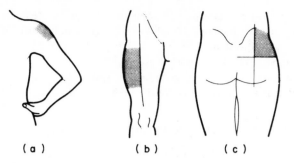

Figure 22.1 The sites for intramuscular injection. (a) Outer aspect of the shoulder; (b) antero-lateral aspect of the thigh; (c) the upper and outer quadrant of the buttock.

The needle should be deep enough to penetrate the muscle without inserting it up to the mount as, should the needle break, there is a better chance of removing it if a piece of the shaft projects above the skin surface (Figure 22.2).

The skin over the selected site is stretched with the left hand. The syringe and needle are held in the right hand and directed at a right angle to the skin surface, then the needle is inserted quickly and firmly deep into the muscle. If a large quantity of drug is to be given by one injection, it must be given very slowly or it will cause pain.

Many drugs may be given by intramuscular injection. Some common examples are penicillin, streptomycin, vitamin B_{12}, Imferon, morphine and atropine.

Sensitization dermatitis

Dermatitis, particularly of the hands, arms and face, may occur in nurses and doctors who come into frequent contact with penicillin, streptomycin or chlorpromazine when giving injections. An investigation into this problem has shown that spraying of the drug occurs when the air

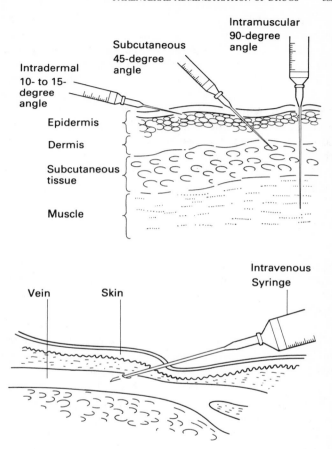

Figure 22.2 Intramuscular, subcutaneous, intradermal and intravenous injections.

is expelled from the syringe and when the needle used for withdrawal of the drug from the container is changed for another needle before giving the injection. Contamination of the hands is also likely if there is a leakage at the junction of the needle and the nozzle of the syringe. In order to minimize the risk of dermatitis it is recommended that the air should be expelled from the syringe into the container before the needle is withdrawn and that the same needle should be used for giving the injection. Care should also be taken to ensure that the needle is firmly attached to the syringe. Wearing plastic gloves gives added protection, and the gloves, hands and arms should be thoroughly washed under running water when the procedure is completed.

Prolonged testing has proved that the needle is not blunted by puncturing the rubber cap of the container.

INTRAVENOUS INJECTION

Nurses who have been given adequate preparation, i.e. who undergo locally approved training, may give drugs that are in common current use via an intravenous line or cannula. The district management team in the UK takes responsibility for this area of practice, which is now part of the extended role of the nurse. Preparation is determined by each hospital or group of hospitals and the nurse will be given a certificate of competence which would be supportive in the case of litigation.

Students and pupil nurses need to be adequately prepared before witnessing the injection of drugs. This again is determined locally.

It is important to note that both trained and student nurses (registered nurses in the UK) participate in this procedure voluntarily and should be under no compulsion to do so if they do not wish to.

Side-effects of drugs given intravenously include anaphylaxis and general and local discomfort to varying degrees. Nursing practice in this and other areas of 'the extended role of the nurse' varies widely throughout the UK and the world. There is no national policy and therefore the nurse must adapt to working for different authorities, obtaining a new certificate of competence from each new employing authority. Problems arise in the use of trial drugs, but these are the sole responsibility of the medical practitioner.

Introduction of drugs or fluid into the circulation by the intravenous route is performed by the doctor.

The usual reasons for using this route are as follows.

1. When a very quick action is required in an emergency.
2. When the drug used would be irritating to the tissues if given intramuscularly or hypodermically, e.g. arsenical preparations.
3. When it is desired to introduce a drug into the circulation for diagnostic purposes, e.g. the various radioopaque media used in X-ray examinations, such as pyelography and angiography.
4. When it is desired to produce local clotting in the treatment of varicose veins.

Intravenous injection is also used as a route for the administration of anaesthetics.

The usual site for the injection is one of the large superficial veins on the front of the elbow.

Note. When large amounts of fluid are to be administered intravenously, this is termed an infusion.

Requirements

- The drug for injection
- Sterile 10- or 20-ml syringe and needles
- Tourniquet or a sphygmomanometer
- Waterproof pillow to support the patient's arm
- Sterile swabs and a sterile towel
- Ether, surgical spirit or cetrimide

- Small adhesive dressing
- Disposal bag for dirty swabs
- Sterile disposable gloves

The skin should be cleaned round the site of the injection, and the tourniquet or the cuff of the sphygmomanometer placed round the arm well above the elbow and then tightened or inflated sufficiently to distend the veins. The cuff of the sphygmomanometer is more convenient than a tourniquet, as it is easier to regulate the pressure so that the venous, but not the arterial, circulation is stopped. Also the wide cuff of the sphygmomanometer is more comfortable for the patient than a narrow rubber tourniquet.

The patient, if able to do so, may help by opening and closing his fist several times.

The nurse will be required to assist by steadying the patient's arm while the needle is being inserted and by releasing the tourniquet or deflating the cuff when the needle is in the vein and before the drug is injected. It is important that the patient should be 'talked through' the procedure, and the nurse should do this if the doctor does not.

23 Infusions

An infusion allows fluid to be administered slowly over long periods of time directly into a tissue or a cavity of the body. The apparatus used incorporates a 'drip' chamber which slows the flow of fluid, the flow being maintained by gravity. A gate clip, attached on the outside of the tubing, is used to compress the tubing and, by adjusting the screw, can be used to slow the flow into discrete drops, regulated to a prescribed number per minute.

The tissues and cavities into which fluid may be given thus are:

1. The venous system
2. The stomach (milk feed)
3. The rectum (administration of some drugs)
4. The bladder (bladder washout and tidal drainage)
5. The peritoneum (peritoneal dialysis)
6. The extradural space (epidural analgesia).

Principles of administration

1. The apparatus should be completely filled with fluid, to exclude all air, before it is attached to the needle or catheter.
2. To prevent air entering the system once it is in use, the tubing should be intact and all connections should be tight.
3. The patient's fluid intake and output should be recorded.

4. With the exception of the stomach and rectal infusions, the apparatus and fluid must be sterile, to prevent microorganisms from gaining access to the body.

INTRAVENOUS INFUSION

Reasons for administering intravenous fluids are as follows.

1. For the replacement or maintenance of fluid volume when the gastrointestinal route is inadequate or cannot be used.
2. To control electrolyte balance when normal physiological mechanisms are inadequate.
3. For rapid and certain delivery of medication when oral, subcutaneous or intramuscular routes are inadequate or unsuitable.
4. For giving nutritious substances when the patient cannot or should not absorb nutrients through the gastrointestinal tract.

Many different fluids may be administered by intravenous infusion.

1. Substances to correct or maintain serum electrolyte levels, or to correct dehydration, for example:
    normal (physiological) saline (NaCl 0.9% solution)
    potassium chloride
    calcium lactate
    sodium bicarbonate 1.3−8.4%
    dextrose 4.3%
    NaCl 0.18%
2. Substances to maintain nutrition, when the patient is unable to take nutrients by other routes, for example:
    dextrose solution 10, 20 or 40%
    amino acids

fructose 5, 10, 20 or 40%
intralipid
galactose 5%

3. Substances to maintain blood pressure, for example:
plasma
dextran solution (10% dextran in normal saline or 10% dextran in dextrose).

Note. Dextran solution is commonly used to improve the capillary circulation in shock and burns. It is also used to improve the circulation in thrombosis.

4. As a vehicle for the administration of drugs. Normal saline is the fluid used, and the drugs which may be administered in this way include antibiotics and noradrenaline.

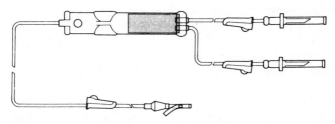

Figure 23.1 Y-type blood/solution administration set.

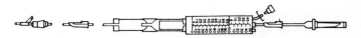

Figure 23.2 Disposable polythene giving set with calibrated chamber.

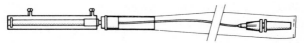

Figure 23.3 An 'intracath'.

Sites which may be used for intravenous infusion are superficial veins over the internal malleolus, over the back of the hand, in the antecubital fossa of the elbow, and scalp veins in babies.

For the purposes of parenteral nutrition (hyperalimentation), highly concentrated hypertonic solutions may be used. In this case, a high-flow major vessel such as the superior vena cava will be used to prevent the risk of phlebitis. The specialist care of such infusions is beyond the scope of this book, and it is usually only entrusted to specially trained nurses.

If necessary, the skin should be shaved before the infusion is set up.

Requirements

- Giving set (no filter is required unless blood is to be given) (Figures 23.1 and 23.2). For children, it should contain a calibrated chamber for greater accuracy.
- The needle, cannula or intracath (Figure 23.3), for insertion into the vein, and an adaptor if necessary
- Gallipot for cleaning lotion or mediswab
- Cotton wool, gauze swabs and towels
- Syringe and needles for local anaesthetic
- Intravenous fluid
- Protective disposable gloves

⎫
⎬ All
⎭ sterile

- The local anaesthetic
- A drip stand
- Sphygmomanometer
- Pillow with a waterproof cover
- Adhesive tape
- Opsite
- The prescribed fluid. This must be checked before

administration to ascertain that is the correct solution at the prescribed strength. PVC and polyethylene containers should be checked before use to ensure that there is no puncture present. Liquids should be inspected to ensure they are absolutely clear and there is no cloudiness or particulate contamination.

- Splint and bandage
- Bandage scissors
- Cut-down set. Very rarely, the venous system may be collapsed, and the skin will have to be incised and the vein exposed in order to puncture it. In this case a 'cut-down' set is used, containing:

  scalpel and blade

  two curved blunt hooks

  an aneurysm needle and thread size 60 or catgut size 00

  a cannula

  one pair each of: toothed and non-toothed dissecting forceps

  needle, needle holder and skin suture

  two pairs of fine artery forceps

  syringe, needle and local anaesthetic.

  (The apparatus will usually be supplied in a 'cut-down' pack).

Method of setting up the infusion

1. The procedure and the reasons for it must be carefully explained to the patient, since his cooperation will be needed in keeping the arm still whilst it is in progress. Information should be carefully selected so the patient is told what he needs to do to help and what the procedure will feel like. He shoud be offered a urinal or bedpan and be made comfortable before it starts.
2. The connector needle at the upper end of the giving set is exposed and inserted into the container of intra-

venous fluid. Air entry must be provided for, if the container is not collapsible. If an air entry tube is an integral part of the giving set, it must be clamped off if the fluid is in a collapsible container. The container must be held upright whilst the connector needle is inserted.

3. The container of fluid is hung on the drip stand, and fluid is allowed to drip rapidly so that the apparatus is filled with fluid and all air is excluded. If the container is a plastic one, it can be gently squeezed to start the flow of fluid. The tubing is clamped when all air has been excluded and the needle adaptor should remain covered until it is connected to the needle. Normally, the liquid reservoir should be hung approximately 1 metre above the patient's shoulder.

4. The sphygmomanometer cuff is applied to the limb above the site of the chosen vein and is inflated to the level of the patient's diastolic blood pressure. The skin over the vein is cleaned with antiseptic lotion, and the selected needle or cannula is inserted by the doctor into the vein, having first donned the sterile gloves. Local anaesthetic may be infiltrated into the area before this if the patient is very nervous, or if there is difficulty in getting the needle into the vein. As soon as blood flows from the needle, the sphygmomanometer cuff is released, the giving set is connected to the needle, and the intravenous fluid is dripped in at the prescribed rate.

5. A dressing is placed in position over the needle and the tubing is also strapped to the limb so that small movements do not dislodge the needle by pulling on the tubing. The limb may be splinted. Opsite is probably the dressing of choice as it is impermeable to fluids and organisms but allows good vision of the site as it is transparent.

6. Clear, written instructions as to rate of flow and the fluid to be given should be obtained from the doctor; the fluid chart should be completed and the patient left comfortable.

7. Frequent observations of the patient and of the infusion will be required.

8. The patient should be given careful instructions about the range of activity he is permitted.

9. Checking the rate of flow should be carried out frequently. The desired rate can be calculated by the formula:

$$\frac{\text{ml per unit}}{\text{hours to be taken for 1 unit}} \times \frac{\text{number of drops per ml of giving set}}{\text{number of minutes per hour}}$$

BLOOD TRANSFUSION

Blood is given directly into a vein as described above, but the procedure is called a transfusion when blood is given, and additional precautions are required.

Whole blood is required when the patient has lost a quantity of blood from the body over a short period of time. It may also be administered in anaemia, where there is a deficiency of red blood cells, or it may be given to increase the clotting power of the blood. Special precautions are required when transfusing blood to ensure that the donor blood is compatible with the recipient's blood. In particular, the donor's red blood cells must be unaffected by the recipient's plasma. Incompatibility between the donor and the recipient blood may result in agglutination or clumping of the donor red cells, with consequent danger of blocking capillaries. A further danger is that of haemolysis of the red cells in large quantities, releasing haemoglobin and potassium into the bloodstream.

Investigation has shown that red blood cells may carry an agglutinogen (two major agglutinogens are classified A and B) whilst blood plasma may contain agglutinins which on contact with a red cell carrying the appropriate agglutinogen causes a reaction of that red cell (Table 23.1).

Other antibody—antigen systems may be present, the most important of these being the Rhesus system. About 85% of Europeans carry an antigen, the Rhesus factor, on their red blood cells (these people are called Rhesus positive), whilst the rest of the population do not have this factor (called Rhesus negative). If a Rhesus negative individual is transfused with Rhesus positive blood, antibodies capable of reacting against red blood cells carrying the Rhesus factor may be formed, so that a second or third contact with Rhesus positive blood at a later date may result in some kind of reaction.

Note. Agglutinins to AB agglutinogens are present in the blood without any contact with the agglutinogen, whilst Rhesus antibody is formed as a *result* of contact with Rhesus positive blood.

It is vital that the patient should receive only that blood which is compatible with his own; for this reason, a

Table 23.1 The ABO blood grouping system.

Blood group	Agglutinogen present on red blood cell	Agglutinin present in plasma
A	A	Anti-B
B	B	Anti-A
AB	A and B	None
O	None	Anti-A and anti-B

Note. It is the effect of the recipient's plasma on the donor cells which is important in transfusions.

specimen of the individual's blood is grouped, and cross-matched with a specimen of the blood from the container of donor blood. This means that the two specimens of blood are mixed in the laboratory and their behaviour is observed. The serial numbers of the units of blood which have been cross-matched against the patient's blood are recorded, and these numbers must be checked against the numbers on the unit label, before the blood is administered. Donor blood is marked with the date at which it was collected, and the date beyond which it should not be used. It should be stored at 4–6°C (39–41°F) and should neither be heated nor cooled before use.

Setting up a blood transfusion

The procedure for blood transfusion is very similar to that for setting up an intravenous infusion of other fluids, except that a giving set with a filter must be used. Normal saline is used to start the infusion and then the checked unit of blood is substituted for the saline. Observations of the patient are especially important whilst a blood transfusion is in progress, to detect any complications which may arise.

Complications which may arise during a blood transfusion

Difficulty in maintaining the flow of blood

There are many reasons why the flow of blood might slow or stop; the nurse should be capable of diagnosing the causes, some of which she can deal with, whilst others must be dealt with by the doctor.

1. The veins may go into spasm. Warming the limb may help.
2. The tubing may become kinked, which is easily put right by the nursing staff.

3. The needle may become dislodged, so that its lumen is obliterated by the vein wall, in which case, lifting the mount of the needle to depress the point may be successful.

4. The needle, or tubing, may become blocked by air. If this happens the apparatus should be disconnected from the needle, and the blood should be allowed to run freely through the tubing before it is reconnected again. This should be carried out by a doctor.

5. The needle or tubing may become blocked by blood clot. If it is the tubing which is blocked, it can dealt with as described in (4) above. If it is the needle, then the doctor may attempt to remove the clot by attaching a syringe to the needle and sucking the clot into the syringe. A new needle may have to be inserted.

Overloading of the circulatory system

The introduction of large volumes of blood, or any other fluid, into the bloodstream can give rise to cardiac and respiratory distress as a result of overloading the circulatory system if cardiac or renal function is insufficient. This danger is greatest when large quantities of fluid are rapidly introduced. Signs and symptoms of this complication are: rising pulse rate; rapid, shallow respirations; pain in the chest; and oedema. If this should occur, the transfusion should be stopped and the doctor informed.

Incompatibility reaction

If an incompatibility reaction should occur it will usually do so soon after the transfusion has started. The symptoms are: shivering; rise in temperature; pain in the lumbar region; nausea and vomiting. The transfusion must be stopped immediately. Later jaundice and oliguria may occur.

Allergic reaction

Blood is a very complex liquid and may contain substances to which the patient is hypersensitive. The symptoms may be mild, such as irritation of the skin and urticaria; or severe, with difficulty in breathing, and laryngeal oedema. In the later case, the transfusion must be stopped and the doctor informed. Adrenaline will be given in severe reactions, antihistamines in mild ones.

Febrile reactions

Fever may result from the introduction of contaminants with the blood. This usually occurs some time after the transfusion has been started, or even after it has been completed. Symptoms are of an increase in temperature and pulse rate. If this should occur whilst the transfusion is in progress, the rate should be slowed and the doctor informed.

Thrombosis of the vein

Venous thrombosis is a fairly common complication, and if it is extensive may be very painful for the patient. There may be a rise in systemic temerature. The doctor should be informed, the transfusion may be stopped, and warmth applied to relieve the pain.

Haematoma

A haematoma may form at the site of entry of the needle into the tissues if the needle becomes dislodged from the vein. The transfusion should be stopped and the limb elevated. Hyaluronidase may be infiltrated into the area to help disperse the blood.

Changing the blood bottle or polythene unit

A new unit of blood which has been cross-matched with the patient's blood should be obtained and carefully checked before the previous unit has been completely administered. The fresh unit is taken to the bedside and its number, and the patient's name, are carefully checked to ensure that the blood is correct for this patient. A new unit should be substituted for the old one before the old one is completely empty, but as little blood as possible should be left in the old container, or blood will be wasted. Mix plasma and cells in the new unit by inverting gently. Do not shake. Clamp the tubing of the giving set to stop the flow from the old unit. This unit is then removed from the drip stand, the piercing connector needle is removed from this unit and quickly inserted into the new one. Care should be taken not to contaminate the connector needle. The new unit is then suspended from the drip stand, and the tubing clip adjusted to allow the blood to flow at the prescribed rate.

INFUSION INTO THE STOMACH (MILK DRIP)

Infusion of fluids into the stomach is used rarely, but occasionally milk is administered by this method in severe peptic ulceration. The milk is placed in a vacuum flask, suspended from a drip stand, and is administered by means of an infusion set which is connected to an oesophageal or Ryle's tube, passed into the stomach. The end of the tube is strapped into position on the patient's cheek. As with all infusions, a fluid balance chart should be maintained, the rate should be observed, and regulated as prescribed. All air should be excluded from the apparatus. (For method of passing tube into the stomach, and checking its position, see Chapter 7.)

RECTAL INFUSION

Rectal infusion is rarely used, but drug solutions or substances to be retained in the rectum for some time before being returned might be given by this method, e.g. olive oil, cortisone solution, magnesium sulphate solution.

A cleansing enema may be administered before setting up the infusion. The apparatus is assembled as for other infusions but it need not be sterile. A small-size rectal catheter is inserted through the anus and the infusion tubing filled with the liquid to be administered is connected to the catheter, and the rate adjusted.

BLADDER WASHOUT AND TIDAL DRAINAGE

The basic apparatus used for intravenous infusion may be modified to allow sterile solutions to drip slowly into the bladder through a self-retaining catheter. For tidal drainage a Y connection should be inserted between the infusion tubing and tubing from the catheter, to allow drainage tubing to be looped up before emptying into a urine container, syphonage of the bladder contents then occurs when the bladder has filled. (For bladder washout see Chapter 24.)

24 Washouts

A body cavity may be washed out as a method of removing or diluting secretions or other contents, and cleaning the area. Areas which may be washed out include the stomach, the rectum, bladder, ear and vagina. Usually, washouts are carried out by the nursing staff. Bladder and vaginal irrigations are sterile procedures, whilst stomach and rectal washout and ear syringing are not.

As with all procedures which the patient undergoes, information-giving is an important function of the nurse. Before the procedure the patient needs to know the following:

1. The purpose of the procedure.
2. The sequence in which the procedure will be carried out.
3. Approximately how long the procedure will last.
4. What each part of the procedure will feel like. (The nurse can collect this information from patients who have already been through the procedure.)
5. How the patient can cope, in terms of the best position to adopt, relaxation methods, deep breathing, distraction, etc.
6. Any after-effects of the procedure.

This information should be given beforehand in terms the patient will understand and the patient should also be kept fully informed throughout the procedure. Frequent reference may be made to the knowledge already possessed by the patient.

STOMACH WASHOUT, RECTAL WASHOUT

Requirements

Common to both procedures

- Length of tubing
- Tubing clip
- Connector for tubing and catheter or oesophageal tube
- Lubricant
- Swabs
- Jug containing washout solution at 37.5°C (99.5°F)
- Lotion thermometer
- Irrigating can or funnel
- Litre measure
- Container for soiled swabs
- Polythene sheets to protect bed and floor
- Pail to receive returned fluid
- Water, normal saline or sodium bicarbonate solution 1:160
- Disposable protective gloves

For rectal washout only

- Rectal tube or catheter size 14 English gauge

For stomach washout only

- Oesophageal tube, size 18 (English gauge), 22 (French gauge)
- Mouthwash if patient is conscious
- Postanaesthetic instruments if patient is unconscious

Stomach washout

Stomach washout may be required in cases of poisoning, to remove all traces of poison from the stomach. A large-bore oesophageal tube is passed, orally. The patient may be in a semi-prone or prone position during the washout, especially if loss of consciousness has occurred. The contents of the stomach are completely removed and kept for examination. The stomach is then washed out using an appropriate solution, such as sodium bicarbonate solution. Sometimes the washout fluid is required for analysis.

Stomach washout may also be carried out in gastritis, pyloric stenosis and preoperatively.

Rectal washout

Rectal washout may be carried out to remove faeces, or to prepare the area before a barium enema or operation. The procedure is continued until the fluid is returned clear.

Syphonage as a method of washout

In the case of both stomach and rectal washout, syphonage can be used as a method of removing the fluid from the organ when once it has been run in. A length of rubber tubing and a funnel should be attached to the tube which is passed into the cavity. The bed and floor should be well protected with polythene sheeting, and a bucket should be placed on the floor to receive the washings. The procedure for passing the tube is different in each case.

Passing the rectal tube

It is important not to allow air into the rectum as it is most uncomfortable for the patient and interferes with syphonage. The apparatus should be completely filled with the washout fluid at the correct temperature and clipped off when all air has been excluded. The rectal tube is then lubricated and passed for 10 cm into the rectum, with the patient in the left lateral position. Approximately 500 ml of fluid is allowed to run in, keeping the funnel filled at all times, so that air does not get into the apparatus. Whilst there is still some fluid in the funnel it is quickly inverted over the bucket and the fluid is allowed to run out. This is repeated until the fluid is returned clear. Both the quantity of fluid introduced and that returned should be measured to check that all fluid is returned.

Passing the stomach tube

The stomach tube is passed in the usual way (see Chapter 7). A check is made that the tube is in the stomach and the stomach contents are aspirated. Fluid is then run in through the funnel and tubing, and syphoned out again, as described above. Only 250 ml of fluid should be run into the stomach at a time.

Other methods of washout

It is possible to carry out a stomach washout with a 50-ml syringe, using the barrel as a funnel to allow the fluid to run in, and then using the piston to aspirate the fluid back.

An alternative method of rectal washout is to allow 500 ml of fluid to run in to the rectum and then to allow the patient to pass the fluid back into a bedpan, commode or lavatory before further fluid is run in.

BLADDER WASHOUT

Bladder washout may be performed after operations in the vicinity of the bladder, such as prostatectomy. An indwelling catheter will have been inserted and connected to a urine drainage bag. Great care should be taken to avoid the introduction of microorganisms into the bladder during this procedure.

Requirements

An intravenous infusion set is connected by a Y or T connection to a piece of tubing from the catheter on the one hand, and a piece of tubing leading to the urine bag on the other. All tubing and connections must be sterile. The infusion set is inserted into a bottle of normal saline 0.9% solution, suspended from a drip stand. All air must be excluded from the apparatus by filling it with the saline before it is connected to the catheter. Spencer Wells forceps, or gate clips, are used as clamps.

To irrigate the bladder

The tubing leading from the catheter to the urine bag is clamped off and a small measured quantity of the normal saline is allowed to drip into the bladder. The tubing leading from the normal saline bottle is then clamped, the other clamp removed, and the irrigating fluid flows out into the urine drainage bag. This can be repeated as frequently as necessary.

25 Diagnostic X-ray procedures

Some body tissues (bone for example) have a greater density than others, and throw a shadow on X-ray which allows their structure to be seen. Air and other gases, which are less dense than body tissue, also show up on X-ray, so when present within an organ may show up that organ. Air, present within the lungs, enables X-rays of the chest to be helpful in diagnosing disorders of the lungs and heart. Where tissues are of a uniform density, however, an individual tissue cannot be seen on X-ray and some kind of 'contrast' medium may have to be used to outline the organ. Contrast media usually contain iodine, but barium or air may be used for this purpose.

STRAIGHT X-RAYS

X-rays in which no contrast medium is introduced are called straight X-rays, and are useful mainly in examination of bony structures, to show up thoracic structures, and to examine the abdomen since there may be gas present in the intestine. Any structure in which calcification has taken place will also show up on straight X-rays. Thus, gall stones, or kidney stones may be seen, or the pineal body in an adult when straight skull X-rays are taken . A great deal of information can be obtained from a straight X-ray by a radiologist, who is trained to identify structures and their abnormalities.

Preparation of the patient before X-ray

In a pilot study to investigate the incidents which affected the anxiety level of a sample of patients in medical wards, Wilson-Barnett (1977) found that anxiety increased before and after an X-ray examination. She found that such anxiety could be reduced by giving the patient information about the preparation for the X-ray, the procedure in the X-ray department and any after effects.

General explanation to any patient going for an X-ray should include the following information.

They may have to sit and wait whilst the X-rays are developed, and therefore it is a good idea to take a book. Shoes and socks may be worn. X-ray rooms are rather dark and the equipment is large and may seem noisy. Patients may be asked to hold their breath whilst the picture is taken but this lasts only a second or so. Whilst an occasional single X-ray is absolutely harmless, the effect is cumulative and so staff who work with X-ray machines the whole time wear protective aprons.

More detailed explanation of the procedure is required for special X-rays (see below). Ill, unconscious and nervous adults should be accompanied by a nurse, and children must always be accompanied, preferably by their mothers. The patient should also be accompanied by a nurse if there is an intravenous infusion or any other technical procedure in progress.

Metal objects, such as brassière fastenings, buttons, hairgrips, zips, show up on X-ray, so the part to be X-rayed must be free of these objects. It is far more satisfactory if a patient wears a plain cotton gown or pyjamas with tapes to fasten them. Elastoplast, kaolin and plaster of Paris show up on X-ray.

SPECIAL X-RAYS

These are X-rays in which some contrast medium is used. Preparation of the patient before the X-ray, or special nursing care or observation afterwards, may be necessary. Since preparation and after-care may vary in detail in different hospitals, only a broad outline is given below.

Information-giving before special X-rays

Reference has been made to Wilson-Barnett's work (1977, 1978) showing an increase in anxiety amongst a sample of patients prior to special X-rays. This anxiety was particularly great amongst patients undergoing barium enema. Furthermore, a group of patients given information prior to barium enema showed significantly lower anxiety than a control group. Such findings have since been confirmed in relation to other special X-rays. Researchers emphasized, in particular, how important it is to give the information beforehand about the sensations the patient will experience during a special X-ray. This is especially so since the patient will probably be left alone during the taking of the films, in a room which may be darkened. This reduces the total sensory stimulation and therefore any sensation experienced due to previous medical or nursing intervention such as an enema will feel greater in contrast and will be particularly frightening.

In order to give helpful information to the patient, nursing staff will need to understand very clearly the following:

1. The procedure for each special X-ray.
2. How the patient should be prepared.
3. What will happen in the X-ray department.

Other information needed for transmission to the patient includes:

4. The nature of the sensations experienced as a result of the injection or instillation of contrast media.
5. Any tilting of the X-ray table or other unusual positions.
6. Methods which the patient can use which help coping.
7. Any after-effects of the X-ray.

Clearly the role of nurses employed within the X-ray department is very important in giving this information to those patients undergoing special X-ray as out-patients. Equally the ward nurse's role is important for in-patients. Within the ward the information can be given in a phased way to be maximally effective.

Examination of the renal tract

There are two ways in which contrast medium may be introduced into the renal tract:

1. By *intravenous injection* (intravenous pyelogram): the iodine compound is excreted from the blood by the kidney and, provided the kidney is functioning normally, the contrast medium becomes concentrated in the urine, outlining the renal tract. It can be seen that some indication of renal function as well as structural detail is obtained by this method.
2. By *retrograde pyelogram*: a cystoscope is passed into the bladder, and a catheter is passed into the ureter of the kidney to be examined. The contrast medium is then injected through this ureteric catheter into the kidney.

Preparation for renal X-ray

Faeces or gas in the intestine obscure the kidney shadow, so the aim of preparation is to prevent either from accumulating. An aperient, e.g. Dulcolax, may be given 36–48 hours before the X-ray is due, and the diet should be adjusted to avoid flatus- or bulk-producing foods. (A low residue diet is given). If at all possible, the patient should be walking about as this helps peristalsis. No food or drink should be given from midnight on the day of the X-ray.

Examination of the gall bladder

Cholecystogram

A contrast medium taken by mouth is absorbed from the intestinal tract and becomes concentrated in the gall bladder, outlining it on X-ray. The procedure is called a cholecystogram. As with renal X-rays, the gall bladder picture can become obscured if faeces or flatus are present in the intestine. Thus an aperient and a low residue diet are given, as described above. The evening before the X-ray, the prescribed radio-opaque substance is given orally to the patient, and following this he should either have nothing by mouth until the X-rays are taken, or water only may be given. When a picture of the gall bladder has been obtained, a fatty meal, or drink, may be given in the X-ray department to stimulate the emptying of the gall bladder, before further films are taken.

Angiography of the gall bladder and bile ducts

Intravenous Biligrafin may be given to be concentrated in the bile to outline the gall bladder. The preparation for this is exactly as for a cholecystogram except that the oral dose of contrast medium is omitted.

If the bile ducts are to be outlined after the gall bladder has been removed, the investigation is called a cholangiogram, and the procedure is as for cholecystography, but no fatty meal is given in X-ray.

Biligrafin may be injected into the T-tube inserted into the common bile duct at cholecystectomy or before the T-tube is removed, about 12 to 14 days postoperatively. The only preparation here is that the T-tube is usually clamped some hours before the injection is made and X-ray pictures are taken.

Examination of the alimentary tract

The contrast medium used for outlining the alimentary tract is barium sulphate and this may be given orally as a suspension (barium meal) or rectally (barium enema).

Barium meal

Medicines containing bismuth must be omitted for 3 days before the X-ray and no aperient should be given within 24 hours of the X-ray. Nothing should be given by mouth for 6 hours prior to the barium meal. The barium is administered as approximately 250 ml of dense cold liquid with a synthetic fruity type of flavour. When the barium has been drunk, its progress through the alimentary tract may be followed by taking X-rays at intervals. This is one X-ray examination in which the patient may be moved into one of several positions, e.g. from side to side, and he should be warned about this. Food is allowed once the stomach is empty of barium, but aperients, antacids and enemas must be avoided until the X-ray films are complete.

Barium enema

The bowel should be empty for a barium enema. A faecal softener may be administered by mouth, some days before the X-ray, and this is followed by a mild aperient, such as Dulcolax. A low residue diet is given.

The evening before the X-ray, an evacuant enema is administered and this is followed by a rectal washout in the morning, before the patient goes to X-ray. Barium sulphate solution is administered as a retention enema in X-ray. Obviously, careful explanations must be given to the patient.

Examination of the bronchi

By injecting opaque medium into the respiratory tract, the bronchi and their branches are outlined on X-ray. The X-ray medium may be inserted over the back of the throat, or by means of a bronchoscope.

Preparation of the patient includes intensive chest physiotherapy and starvation for the 6 hours immediately before the X-ray, to prevent vomiting. A mild sedative and a drug which will inhibit bronchial secretions may be given within 1 hour of the examination. A local anaesthetic will be given to the throat, so the patient must not be allowed to eat and drink until the effects of this have worn off after the X-ray (i.e. not until the cough reflex returns).

Intensive chest physiotherapy must be given after the X-ray to remove the contrast medium from the respiratory tract.

Examination of the central nervous system

Ventriculography

Air is inserted into the lateral ventricles of the brain. By careful positioning of the patient on the X-ray table, the air can be made to show the shape and position of the lateral and third ventricles. In order to inject the air into the ventricles, burr holes must be made in the skull in the postparietal region. This involves an operation which may be carried out under local or general anaesthetic. Pre-operatively the postparietal scalp area must be shaved, and the patient is prepared as for a general anaesthetic, even if the procedure is to be done under a local anaesthetic, since operation may be urgent if the films show up some abnormality. After ventriculography, the patient must be observed carefully, particular note being taken of conscious level, limb movements, pupillary reflexes, pulse rate, respiratory rate and blood pressure.

Increasingly, District Health Authorities are acquiring C.T. Scanners. These are generally used for non-invasive techniques. They allow diagnosis without the use of many invasive procedures such as ventriculography.

Examination of the cardiovascular system

Cardiac catheterization

This is carried out to measure the blood pressure in the chambers of the heart, and to withdraw samples of blood from the chambers to estimate its oxygen content. Defects of the heart can be shown using this technique. A long opaque catheter is introduced into a vein in the right arm and is passed through the venous system into the right atrium, right ventricle, and pulmonary artery. Its progress can be watched on a television screen (Figures 25.1 and 25.2).

A nurse should accompany a patient who is having this procedure carried out. A general anaesthetic is not usually given as it lowers the pressures within the heart.

Angiography

Radio-opaque contrast medium is injected through the cardiac catheter. No special preparation of the patient is

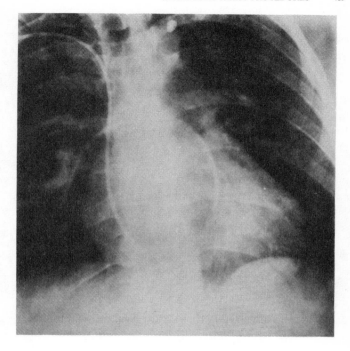

Figure 25.1 Cardiac catheterization of the normal heart.

needed. An adult is given a sedative before going to X-ray. A child may require a general anaesthetic.

Arteriography

An opaque medium is injected directly into arteries to outline the arterial wall, or the blood supply to a particular area.

Femoral arteriography. This may be used to outline the blood supply to the lower limbs, the placenta or the

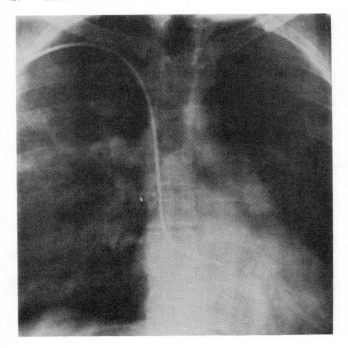

Figure 25.2 Cardiac catheterization of heart with atrial septal defect.

kidneys (Figure 25.3). The investigation is carried out under general anaesthetic and the patient must be prepared accordingly. The area near the femoral artery must be shaved (pubic shave). A guide wire is introduced into the artery and a catheter is fed over it to the required position. When the guide wire has been withdrawn, the catheter can be used to inject the contrast medium.

Carotid arteriography. This is used to demonstrate the cerebral blood vessels and is carried out under general

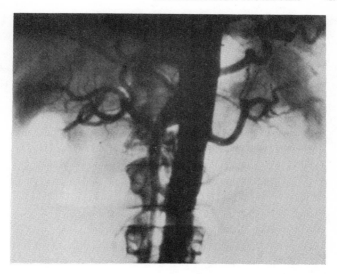

Figure 25.3 Renal arteriogram.

anaesthetic. If it should be carried out under local anaesthetic, sedative drugs are given to the patient beforehand (Figure 25.4). After the investigation, the site of injection in the neck must be observed carefully to note any haematoma formation which could lead to asphyxia. If this should happen, a tracheostomy would be required as an emergency. The patient's conscious level, limb movements, pupillary reflexes, pulse rate, respiratory rate and blood pressure must be observed as well.

Subclavian arteriography. Intracranial blood vessels supplied by the vertebral arteries may be outlined by subclavian arteriography. It is carried out under general anaesthetic. Postoperatively, the patient must be observed

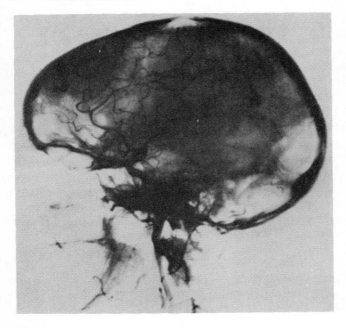

Figure 25.4 Carotid arteriogram.

as described above, but it is particularly important to watch for signs of respiratory distress, since the subclavian artery is very near to the pleural cavity.

26   Bandaging

Although a number of methods can be used to secure surgical dressings, there are still occasions when a properly applied bandage is the best way of retaining a dressing in position. Bandages are also used to fix splints, to apply pressure in order to stop bleeding, and to give support and prevent swelling, as in the treatment of a sprained ankle.

Types of bandages

- *Roller*: these may be several metres long and up to 15 cm in width. The parts of the bandage are known as the initial end, the drum and the tail.
- *Triangular*: 1.5 m^2 of material cut diagonally makes two bandages.
- *Many-tailed*: tails 10 cm wide, the length varies from 1.2 m to 2 m, width of the back 15 to 20 cm. These measurements are for chest and abdominal bandages.
- *Tubular gauze*: for limb and head bandages.
- *Elastic net*: can be used to secure dressings in all parts of the body. It is available in many different sizes.

Materials used for bandages

- *Open-weave cotton*: light and inexpensive, but does not give much support, and the edges fray unless the selvedge edge type is used.
- *Calico*: harsh and inelastic, but firm; useful for slings and for applying splints.

- *Crêpe*: comfortable and gives good support, elastic and easy to apply, expensive but washable.

Roller bandages (Figure 26.1)

Rules for applying roller bandages

1. Stand in front of the part to be bandaged.
2. Pad the axilla or groin when bandaging near these parts.
3. Start with an oblique turn.
4. Bandage from below upwards, and from within outwards.
5. Apply the bandage with firm even pressure throughout.
6. Cover two-thirds of the previous turn of the bandage leaving one-third uncovered.
7. The drum of the bandage must be held uppermost.
8. Reverse on the outside of the limb.
9. Finish with a spiral turn, turning in the end of the bandage and securing it with a safety-pin arranged with point uppermost or with a small strip of adhesive tape.

Points to remember

1. The comfort of the patient is the first consideration

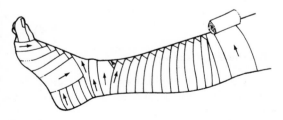

Figure 26.1 Applying a roller bandage (figure-of-eight and reversed turn bandaging).

except when arresting haemorrhage or correcting deformity.

2. Two skin surfaces should not be allowed to lie in contact under the bandage; if this point is not attended to, the skin is liable to become moist and sore.

3. The position of the part: place the limb in the position in which it can most easily be maintained by the patient without strain.

4. Neatness and economy of bandage should be considered, but the bandage must fulfil its purpose and must always completely cover the dressing.

Stump bandaging (Figure 26.2)

The stump is bandaged in order to prevent oedema, to encourage good venous return and tone up flabby tissue, to accustom the stump to being constantly covered, and to prevent an adductor roll of flesh in the groin. Crêpe or Rayolast bandage is used, 15 cm wide for above knee, or 10 cm wide for below knee stumps.

Start by placing the end of the bandage in the centre of the upper side of the stump at the level of the inguinal ligament. Then carry the bandage down and over the stump to the same position on the underside; ask the patient to hold the loops in position with his fingers. Continue to carry the bandage to and fro over the stump, in turn covering the lateral side and then the medial side. Fix the loops with a diagonal turn from the outside top to the inside bottom of the stump, and make a second diagonal turn in the opposite direction. Make straight turns round the stump, making sure it passes high into the groin, pass it round the abdomen and cross on the iliac crest. Make sure the stump is not pulled into flexion. The bandage should not be uncomfortably tight but should exert slight tension on the stump.

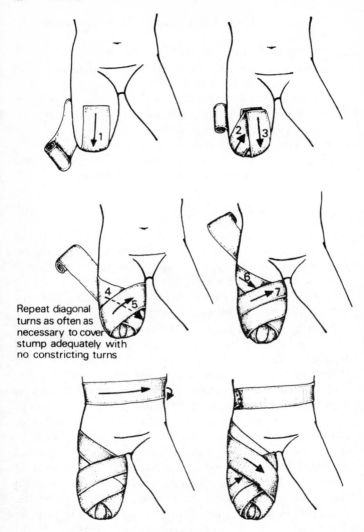

Repeat diagonal turns as often as necessary to cover stump adequately with no constricting turns

Figure 26.2   Different stages in stump bandaging.

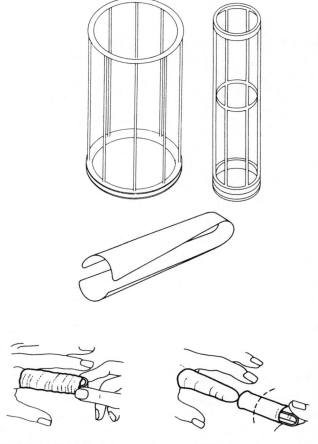

Figure 26.3 Tubular gauze bandages. (a) Tubular gauze applicators; tubular gauze gathered on to a finger size applicator and placed over the finger; (c) applicator withdrawn and twisted at top of finger.

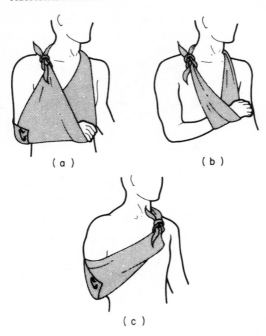

Figure 26.4   Arm slings. (a) Large arm sling; (b) narrow arm sling; (c) St John arm sling.

Tubular gauze bandages

Tubular gauze bandages are a comfortable, neat and efficient method of retaining dressings in position. The gauze is made in various dimensions suitable for many purposes. For bandaging limbs, wire cage applicators on which the gauze is stretched are used (Figure 26.3). The applicator is passed over the part to be bandaged and then withdrawn leaving a layer of gauze covering the area. This procedure is repeated to give as many layers as are necessary covering the part.

It is claimed that a great degree of control over the tension of the bandage is possible with this method and also that the bandage will retain its position better than the usual roller bandage. Many casualty departments find that tubular gauze is particularly useful for finger dressings and that the light, neat bandage is greatly appreciated by patients. Tubular gauze also makes a satisfactory and comfortable head bandage.

Triangular bandages

Triangular calico bandages are used as slings and as first aid bandages (Figure 26.4). They are also useful for holding dressings in position on areas where roller bandages would be difficult to apply or would be heavy and cumbrous.

PART V: Continuity of care

27 Reporting and record keeping

Since neither in the community nor in hospital is any nurse on duty for 24 hours a day 7 days a week, careful record keeping and reporting is needed to ensure continuity of care for patients. Individualized nursing history-taking, assessment, and written care planning help in the maintenance of continuity of care. So does the concept of primary nursing. It will be recalled that the primary nurse has continuing responsibility for the patient, and can give advice to associate nurses by telephone, as and when necessary.

Care plans are primary health documents. This means they will be held in the patient's case notes and retained within medical records for a maximum of 20 years. They form legal records.

Whilst the community and hospital situations have much in common there are some distinctions to be made about actual practice regarding record keeping in the two different settings.

Community nursing

As in hospital, the basic tool for prescribing and recording care is the nursing care plan. This is retained within the patient's home and forms the ongoing record ensuring continuity of care, since less highly qualified nurses and informal carers participate in care as well as the qualified community nurse, who acts as the primary nurse.

In addition to the care plan, the qualified district nurse

will also maintain a card system for each person who forms part of the caseload. Cards are held in the health centre base of the nurse. They record the treatment or care ordered, and any changes to the treatment or care. In addition to these two records, the health authority also requires information about patients receiving care from the district nursing service. This is currently fairly simple factual information. It is frequently fed into a hand-held computer by the nurse at the time of visiting the patient. Later, the information is transferred through a terminal to the main frame computer to be transmitted to the regional health authority.

Continuity between community and hospital

Ideally, care plans would accompany patients from the community to hospital, and back again when the patient is discharged. This would ensure true continuity of care. However, this procedure rarely appears to happen in practice. Therefore it is usual, for a summary of the care plan to be used to transmit information about care between community and hospital and again between hospital and community. Speed in preparing and sending these summaries is crucial to continuity. Unfortunately they may be delayed whilst waiting for typing or over weekends.

Community liaison nurses

Another way of ensuring continuity of care is the use of a community liaison nurse. Ideally, of course, the patient's own primary community nurse would liaise whilst one of the patients from the caseload was in hospital. This may not happen due to heavy caseloads and the distance of the hospital from the community nurse's 'patch'. Instead, special community liaison nurses may be appointed by a district health authority to liaise between hospital and community nurses and ensure continuity of care.

Another way in which continuity of care can be enhanced is by the use of clinical specialist nurses, such as the continence adviser, stomatherapist, diabetic specialist nurse, or a terminal care advisory team. These specialists may advise other nurses about care or may advise patients directly. In any case they usually deliver their services both within hospital and the community.

Hospital nursing

A hospital patient requires observation, nursing care and treatment throughout each 24-hour period. If his care was the complete responsibility of one nurse during a shift, the patient would be cared for by at least three nurses during 24 hours. This means that many different nurses may participate in the observation, nursing care and treatment of any one patient during each day of his stay in hospital. Continuity of care and the pursuit of common objectives in treatment depend upon effective communication between different members of staff, accurate record keeping, clear and objective reporting and precise verbal and written instructions.

THE IMPORTANCE OF COMMUNICATION

The permanent staff of a ward form a social group which has a system of values and norms of its own. Patients and student nurses form temporary members of this social group. They frequently need to infer the group norms and values in a brief period of time in order to 'fit in'. Informal communication is an important vehicle for transmitting norms and values. Revans (1964) found that the morale of ward staff affected patient's recovery. In turn, the morale of staff depended upon communication.

Ward communications in three hospitals were studied by Lelean (1973). She classified communication as formal or informal. Formal communication was defined as those channels and methods of communicaiton which have been consciously and deliberately established (e.g. report books, Kardex, routine verbal reporting sessions). Informal communication was defined as any method of communication which does not form part of the formal system. It is built round the social relationships of individual members of the organization (e.g. gossip, social conversation, impromptu instructions).

The content of informal communication was not observed. Attention was focused on the ward sister and a record was kept of persons which whom the sister communicated and the length of time spent in each communication. Lelean found that whilst the sister spent an average total of 40 to 50 minutes in communication with doctors during the 8 a.m. to 12 noon period of observation, the average total time the sister spent in informal communication with nurses in the same period was 37 to 40 min, less than the time spent communicating with the doctors. For nurses, the importance of formal communication in exchanging information about patients is emphasized by this finding, together with the observation that the more junior the nurse, the less likely it was that the sister spent time communicating with her. On 80% of the days when a first-year student nurse was on duty during the 4 hours, the sister spoke to her for less than 2 minutes. From this, the inference can be drawn that the more junior a nurse, the more careful she should be in ensuring that she understands what is said to her in the formal reporting session about each patient and what is required of her in relation to the nursing care of each patient. Each nurse must also ensure that she knows where she may seek information. Primary nursing may help to overcome such problems.

Formal communications

Formal communication about patients takes two main forms.

1. Records of the patient's history, progress and care given.
2. Instructions for treatment and care (the nursing care plan).

These communications should be written so that they form permanent (and legal) records, but are usually the subject of verbal communication as well.

Records of the patient's history and progress

There are many of these records and they include the doctor's case notes, the temperature, pulse and respiration chart, fluid balance chart, anaesthetic record, consent form, and laboratory reports, as well as the formal nursing care plan and report. Accurate completion of temperature, pulse and respiration and fluid balance charts is mentioned in Chapters 18 and 19.

The nursing report is another document which should be completed neatly, accurately and conscientiously. It forms a legal record of both the care and treatment a patient received in hospital and of his progress. Too often, the nursing report may be a poor record of nursing care, as it may be dominated by details of medical treatment, with little attention being paid to such items as the fact that the patient was turned 2-hourly, or that 4-hourly observations were made.

Most hospitals use either a Kardex system or special sheets of A4 (297 × 210 mm) paper which can then be filed into the patient's case notes when he is discharged, along with all other primary documents pertaining to the patient's stay in hospital.

Information obtained from the patient on admission is documented on the first sheet of the nursing care plan and report. This includes the patient's name, address, age, religion, next of kin and diagnosis. The first entry should report the date and time of the patient's admission, and the mode of transport to the hospital. This gives an idea of mobility levels. Next, the history of the illness should be documented and any observations about the patient's condition on admission (see Chapters 6 and 18), including information of relevance to nursing care (e.g. the state of the skin and mouth, the risk category with respect to pressure sores, the nutritional state). The social adjustment to hospital should also be reported (e.g. whether the patient is anxious, relaxed, apprehensive, or settled well; if he was upset, emotional, quiet or garrulous). It is always better to report actual observations than an interpretation of the observations.

Once the admission report has been written, any important event which occurs (e.g. a dressing, the detection of a red area of skin over a pressure area, observations made during an epileptic fit, a blood transfusion) should be written into the report as soon as possible after the occurrence. Such reports are signed at the end of each shift by the nurse in charge of the patient's care. Each patient should be reported on at the end of each shift to indicate his condition and progress during the shift. A nurse who signs a report must ensure that what is written is accurate, as she is legally responsible for the record which she has signed.

Handwriting should be legible, abbreviations should be avoided and objectivity of reporting should be the aim when writing the report. Each report should be as informative as possible. Phrases such as 'her usual self' will be quite meaningless when used as a record in 2 years' time, or to a new nurse the next day, especially if 'her usual self' has never been described in an earlier report.

Instructions for treatment and care

Written instructions of nursing care on the care plan should be legibly written, frequently revised, and should serve not only as an instruction but also as a record that the care was given and by whom. Previous instructions which are no longer valid should be neatly crossed through and initialled. The instruction should still be clearly readable. Instructions should be very precise and have a clearly understood, unambiguous meaning. It has been found (Lelean, 1973) that instructions, especially those about a patient's mobility, were not consistently understood. Their meaning was context bound in that what a ward sister meant by 'get her up' depended upon the particular patient referred to. Also, the instruction 'up and about' had eight different meanings, and an instruction could have up to three different meanings on the same ward on the same day. This kind of thing makes the delivery of nursing care a very hit-and-miss affair, especially if the nurse receiving the instruction is new to the ward or has just returned from a day off.

An example of an explicit instruction would be as outlined in Figure 27.1.

Further examples of explicit instructions can be seen in the sample care plan in Chapter 4.

Verbal communication

The verbal report has a different function from the written one as it can be used as an opportunity for the exchange of information about patients, for teaching and for questioning about poorly understood terms and instructions.

Patient's name: Mrs Smith

| | Record of care | | |
Instruction	Time up	Time back	Signature
Period up			
To sit out of bed in a chair for			
3½ hours			
Toilet			
To be wheeled to toilet in a			
Sanichair			
Washing			
Provide with a bowl for washing			
herself but feet must be washed			
for patient			
Mobility			
Must be lifted from bed to chair			

Figure 27.1   Example of instructions for treatment and care.

However, it may have disadvantages. These are mainly because of the limitations of human memory. We cannot remember every word that we hear and so the verbal reporting session needs to be supplemented by ready access to written reports and instructions. Sometimes the reporting session may be interrupted and, unless there is always an overlap of shift and the formal report is given at the beginning of each shift, there will have to be at least one nurse who stays to look after patients. Part-time staff may not always start work at the same time as other members of staff. Some wards tape record the verbal report so that nurses may listen later if they have missed the report. This seems a good idea provided the confidentiality of information about patients is respected. Updating of taped reports is important if they are to be useful.

Principles of communication

Several principles should be borne in mind in staff-to-staff communication.

1. Clarity of expression is crucially important, both in speech and writing, so that there is no ambiguity. The meaning should be clear to the recipients whether or not they know the patient concerned.
2. Written records are legal documents and must be accurate.
3. Objective description is better than subjective interpretation.
4. Avoid abbreviations, jargon, and slang expresssions which might not be understood by someone from another hospital or for whom English is a second language.
5. Instructions should be precise so that individuals can carry out the instruction in the way which was intended even though they have never worked on that ward before.

Good records can be used to help continuity of care over day and night shifts, and to compile a report about the patient's hospital care and progress which can be sent to the community nurse on discharge, to be used as a guide for a further plan of nursing care.

28 Discharge of patient: ensuring continuity of care

For some patients, preparation for discharge from hospital may have to start from the moment they are admitted. Problem identification following nursing assessment and history taking may well have shown the importance of teaching the patient skills or knowledge to enable him to cope when returning home on discharge. Teaching objectives and methods then have to be written into the care plan so that the teaching can be carried out throughout the stay in hospital.

There are many diagnostic categories or medical conditions in which patient teaching for discharge assumes an important element in the nursing care plan. Below are some examples of conditions in which teaching is important, together with associated teaching objectives.

Diabetes mellitus

On discharge, the patient should be able to:

1. Draw up the correct dose of insulin, or understand the use of a pen-style device for insulin administration.
2. Choose an appropriate injection site, and understand how to vary the site.
3. Inject himself with insulin.
4. Test urine with Clinitest and Ketostix.
5. Understand the significance of the results of urine testing.

6. Understand the principles of diet and how to ensure that he receives the correct amount of carbohydrate to balance the insulin.

7. Recognize subjectively how it feels (the symptoms) when there is excessive insulin in the body.

8. Know what action to take when experiencing the symptoms of excessive insulin.

9. Understand the reasons for greater than normal care with skin hygiene and care of the feet.

10. Understand potential problems associated with fever or violent exercise.

11. Know principles of balancing diet and insulin when planning to undertake exercise.

12. Be able to test blood for glucose levels.

After colostomy or ileostomy

On discharge, the patient should be able to:

1. Understand principles of controlling the consistency of faecal matter by adjusting the diet; this means understanding which foods are irritant to the gut, which add bulk to the intestinal contents, which slow peristalsis, etc. (also an understanding of the role of fluid intake is important).

2. Clean the skin and protect it from excoriation.

3. Apply and remove a colostomy or ileostomy bag.

4. Know how to dispose of a used bag under home conditions, especially if there is no open fire at home.

5. Know how to deal with the smell, from an ileostomy in particular.

6. Get in touch with patient associations where support and help can be found.

7. Get in touch with the specialist nurse if there is one employed in the area.

8. Understand the different appliances available and how to choose the best one, also how to obtain supplies of appliances and dressings.

After an operation for a hernia

On discharge, the patient should be able to:

1. Lift without causing strain on the muscles involved in the hernia.
2. Understand the necessity to avoid lifting until after the first out-patient appointment.
3. Know how to care for the wound until the sutures have been removed.

Diagnosis of heart failure

On discharge, a patient with a diagnosis of heart failure should be able to:

1. Take his own pulse rate and omit the dose of digoxin if the pulse is lower than 60/minute.
2. Understand the significance of other signs of digoxin accumulation in the body, such as coupling of the pulse beats, nausea, vomiting, visual changes, including changes in colour vision.
3. Know the action to take if there are signs of digoxin accumulation.
4. Understand the importance of taking slow K alongside the diuretic drug.
5. Understand that he will pass a lot of urine after taking the diuretic drug so he can take the drug at the most convenient time to fit daily activities at home.
6. Understand weight changes associated with diuretic drugs.
7. Understand the possible feeling of weakness after taking a diuretic drug.

8. Avoid taking excess salt in the diet.
9. Understand the importance of an adequate fluid intake when taking a diuretic drug to avoid dehydration.

Patient teaching is an element in the nursing care of all patients prior to discharge. Examples have been chosen where teaching plays a particularly important role (diabetes mellitus, ileostomy and colostomy). Two examples are also given where the teaching aspect of nursing is less obvious and may be overlooked (hernia and heart failure). Remember that clinical nurse specialists may be available for referral both in the case of diabetes and for patients with a colostomy or ileostomy.

For patients who have some disability, a nursing assessment, before the discharge date, of the patient's ability to care for himself at home is important. Such assessment would be centred around normal activities of daily living. The patients may be assessed on any of the following items to ensure he can cope at home.

1. Is independent dressing possible?
2. Is there any restriction of movement preventing foot care?
3. Can the patient brush and comb the hair?
4. Is independent walking to the toilet possible?
5. Is the patient fully continent?
6. Can the patient lower himself on to a chair and then get up without help?
7. For how long can the patient stand independently? e.g. 5 minutes, 10 minutes (necessary for activities such as cooking)
8. Is independent feeding possible?
9. Can the patient walk holding a full cup and saucer?
10. Can the patient climb a full flight of stairs?
11. Is mobility sufficient to mount the step of a bus?
12. Can the patient walk carrying shopping?

If the answer to any of these questions is no, then it may be helpful to make a referral to the physiotherapist and occupational therapist. The patient may have therapy to teach him these activities, or it may be useful to get aids made. A home assessment visit by the occupational therapist may be necessary.

Before discharge, most patients need advice about looking after themselves until they feel completely fit again. Such advice may include:

1. How much physical activity the patient should do, together with advice on increasing activity slowly.
2. How and when to take drugs.
3. If certain foods or patent medicines should be avoided since they could interact with prescribed drugs.
4. If he needs to rest in the daytime.
5. When he may return to work.
6. Any possible complications which should be reported to the general practitioner.

Advice should be given about any dietary modification; when sexual activity can be resumed (and if there are any restrictions as to position); the fact that he may feel tired; and how long it is likely to be before he feels completely well again.

Once the discharge date is known, there are certain administrative procedures needed to ensure continuity of care.

If the relatives cannot provide transport for the patient, or if he is being transferred to another hospital whilst still very ill, it will be necessary to order a hospital car or ambulance. Unless the patient is being transported by stretcher, the relatives will be asked to bring in outdoor clothing. The time of discharge must be discussed with relatives to ensure that someone is at home to greet the patient. Any drugs or dressings that will be required should be obtained, and appointments made for the out-patient, physiotherapy or occupational therapy departments, as necessary. When a supply of drugs is given to the patient to take home, a reminder should be given of the times at which they should be taken. It is usual for a final examination to be carried out by the medical staff just before discharge. Any clothing or valuables held by the hospital should be returned to the patient.

Early discharge from hospital is the norm today. This means that community nursing services are more frequently needed than was once the case. Wound dressing, stitch removal and administration of drugs are some of the items of continuing care required. Good communication with the district nurse is essential to ensure continuity of care.

In a report of a survey of recently discharged hospital patients carried out by Skeet (1971), she suggests that the following require urgent attention.

1. Two-way communication between hospital authorities and patients, to include hospital staff receiving information regarding the home conditions and domestic arrangements to which their patients are returning, and patients receiving information and advice concerning their treatment and after-care.
2. Adequate notice of discharge dates to enable patients and their families to make appropriate domestic arrangements in advance.
3. Written instructions to patients on activity, diet, prostheses, effects of drugs and treatment.
4. Adequate staff and equipment to provide a competent clerical service enabling discharge communications to be sent immediately when patients leave hospital.
5. Programmes of after-care planned well in advance of patients' discharge dates and organized in conjunction

with patient's general practitioners and staff of the community services, to provide an unbroken service of nursing and personal care.

The patient's final impression of the hospital will be like the first, a lasting one, and although he will no doubt be anxious to get home, worry may occur about being able to cope without the support and security that having nursing and medical staff constantly available brings. If encouraged to be as independent as possible during the whole of the hospital stay, he will be in a better position to readjust to normal life.

Bibliography

Aggleton P & Chalmers H (1986) *Nursing Models and the Nursing Process*. Basingstoke: Macmillan Education.

Aggleton P & Chalmers H (1990) Nursing models. Model future. *Nursing Times* **86**: 41–43.

Bevan DR (1975) Tracheostomy. *Nursing Times* **71**: 1371.

Bower FL (1977) *The Process of Planning Nursing Care: a Model for Practice* 2nd edn. St Louis: CV Mosby.

Carpenter M (1980) Asylum nursing before 1914: a chapter in the history of labour. In Davis C (ed.) *Rewriting Nursing History*, pp 123–146. London: Croom Helm.

Cartwright A (1964) *Human Relations and Hospital Care*. London: Routledge & Kegan Paul.

Clark J (1985) *The process of health visiting*. PhD Thesis, Polytechnic of the South Bank, London.

Clarke M (1984) Stress and coping: constructs for nursing. *Journal of Advanced Nursing* **9**: pp 3–13.

Coates VE (1982) *An investigation of the nutritional care given by nurses to acute medical patients, and of the influence that ward organisation patterns may have upon that care*. MPhil Dissertation, University of Hull.

Coleman C & Hammen CL (1976) *Contemporary Psychology and Effective Behaviour*. Glenview IL: Scott Foresman.

Corbeil M (1971) Nursing process for a patient with a body image disturbance. *Nursing Clinics of North America* **6**: 156–157.

Coutts LC & Hardy LK (1985) *Teaching for Health*. Edinburgh: Churchill Livingstone.

Devine EC & Cook TD (1986) Clinical and cost saving effects of psychoeducational interventions with surgical patients: A Meta Analysis. *Research in Nursing and Health* **9**: 89–105.

DHSS (1979) *Recommended Daily Amounts of Food, Energy and Nutrients for Groups of People in the United Kingdom*. London: HMSO.

DHSS (1989a) *Working for Patients* (Review of the NHS). London: HMSO.

DHSS (1989b) *Working for Patients*, Education and Training Working Paper 10, HMSO: London.

DHSS (1989c) *Caring for People: Community Care in the Next Decade and Beyond*, Cmnd 849. London: HMSO.

Dingwall R, Rafferty AM & Webster C (1988) *An Introduction to the Social History of Nursing*, London: Routledge.

English National Board for Nursing, Midwifery and Health Visiting (1985) *Professional Education/Training Course: Consultative Paper*. London: ENB.

Glaser BG & Strauss AL (1965) *Awareness of Dying*. Chicago: Aldine.

Gregory J (1978) *Patients' Attitudes to the Hospital Service*, Paper No 5 for the Royal Commission on the National Health Service. London: HMSO.

Gyllensköld K (1982) *Breast Cancer: The Psychological Effects of the Disease and its Treatment*. (Translated by Patricia Crampton.) London: Tavistock Publications.

Hamilton-Smith S (1972) *Nil by Mouth*. London: RCN.

Hayward J (1975) *Information: a Prescription against Pain*. London: HMSO.

Henderson V (1964) The nature of nursing. *American Journal of Nursing* **64**: 63.

Henderson V (1966) *The Nature of Nursing; a Definition and its Implications for Practice, Research and Education*. New York: Macmillan.

Hill GL, Blackett RL, Pickerford IR et al (1977) Malnutrition in surgical patients — an unrecognised problem. *Lancet* i: 689–692.

Holmes TH & Rahe RH (1967) The Social Readjustment Rating Scale. *Journal of Psychosomatic Research* **11**: 213.

Johnson JE, Rice VH, Fuller SS & Endress MP (1978) Sensory information, instruction in coping strategy and recovery from surgery. *Research in Nursing and Health* **1**: 4–17.

Jones D (1975) *Food for Thought*. London. RCN.

Kornfield DS (1979) The hospital environment: its impact on the patient. In Garfield CA (ed.) *Stress and Survival*, pp 154–161. St Louis: CV Mosby.

Kubler Ross E (1969) *On Death and Dying*. New York. Macmillan.

Lazarus RS & Launier R (1978) Stress related transactions between person and environment. In Pervin M & Lewis M (eds) *Perspectives in International Psychology*, pp 287–327. New York: Plenum Press.

Lee PR & Franks PE (1980) Health and disease in the community. In Fry J (ed.) *Primary Care*, pp 3–34. London: Heinemann.

Lelean S (1973) *Ready for Report Nurse?* London: RCN.

Levin LS, Katz, AH & Holst E (1977) *Self-Care? Lay Initiatives in Health*. London: Croom Helm.

Ley P & Spelman MS (1967) *Communicating with the Patient*. St Albans: Staples Press.

Lundman B, Astland K & Norberg A (1988) Tedium among patients with insulin-dependent diabetes mellitis. *Journal Advanced Nursing* **13**: 23–32.

McCaffery M (1979) *Nursing the Patient in Pain* 2nd edn. Philadelphia: Lippincott.

Mayers M (1978) *A Systematic Approach to the Nursing Care Plan* 2nd edn. New York: Appleton-Century-Crofts.

Melia K (1982) Tell it as it is — qualitative methodology and nursing research: understanding the student nurse's world. *Journal of Advanced Nursing* 7: 327.

Menzies I (1961) *The Functioning of Social Systems as a Defence against Anxiety*. London: Tavistock Publication.

Moghissi K & Boore J (1983) Parenteral and Enteral Nutrition for Nurses. London: Heineman

National Advisory Committee on Nutrition Education (1983) *Proposals for Nutritional Guidance for Health Education in Britain*. London: HMSO.

Norris CM (1970) The professional nurse and body image. In Carlson CE (ed.) *Behavioural Concepts and Nursing Intervention*, pp 39–65.

Norton C (1986) *Nursing for Continence*. Beaconsfield: Beaconsfield Publishers Ltd.

Norton D, McLaren R & Exton-Smith AN (1962) *An Investigation of Geriatric Nursing Problems in Hospital*. London: National Corporation for the Care of Old People.

Orem D (1980) *Nursing: Concepts of Practice* 2nd edn. New York: McGraw Hill.

Owen G (1977) *Health Visiting*. London: Baillière Tindall.

Parkes CM (1975) *Bereavement: Study of Grief in Adult Life*. Middlesex: Penguin Books.

Parkes CM (1972) *Bereavement: Studies of Grief in Adult Life*. New York: International Universities Press.

Platt BS, Eddy TP & Pellett PL (1963) *Food in Hospitals*. Oxford: Nuffield Provincial Hospitals Trust.

Quinn S (1980) *Nursing in the European Community*. London: Croom Helm.

Revans RW (1964) *Standards for Morale*. Oxford: Oxford University Press for Nuffield Provincial Hospital Trust.

Riehl JP & Roy C (1980) *Conceptual Models for Nursing Practice* 2nd edn. New York: Appleton-Century-Crofts.

Roberts I (1976) *Discharged from Hospital*. London. RCN.

Roper N, Logan WW & Tierney AJ (1980) *The Elements of Nursing*. Edinburgh: Churchill Livingstone.

Royal College of Nursing (1985) Commission on Nursing Education, *The Education of Nurses: A New Dispensation*. Chairman: Dr Henry Judge, London: RCN.

Royal College of Physicians (1989) *Fractured Neck of Femur: Prevention and Management*. London: RCP.

Scales JT (1975) Pressure on the patient. In *Biomechanics of Tissue Viability and Clinical Applications*. Glasgow: University of

Stratchclyde.

Selye H (1956) The Stress of Life 2nd edn. New York: McGraw-Hill.

Skeet M (1971) *Home from Hospital*. London: Dan Mason Nursing Research Committee.

Smith HS (1974) *Nil by Mouth*. London: RCN.

Spelman MA, Ley P & Jones C (1966) How do we improve doctor–patient communications in our hospitals? *World Hospitals* **2**: 126.

Strauss AL, Corbin J, Fagerhaugh S et al (1984) *Chronic Illness and the Quality of Life* 2nd edn. St Louis: CV Mosby.

United Kingdom Central Council for Nursing, Midwifery and Health Visiting (1986) Project 2000: *A New Preparation for Practice*. London: UKCC.

White R (1978) *Social Change and the Development of the Nursing Profession*. London: Henry Kimpton.

WHO Regional Office for Europe (1986) *Targets for Health for All Implications for Nursing/Midwifery*. Copenhagen: WHO.

Wilson-Barnett J (1977) *Stress in Hospital*. Edinburgh: Churchill Livingstone.

Wilson-Barnett J (1978) Patients' emotional responses to barium X-rays. *Journal of Advanced Nursing* **3**: 37–46.

Wilson-Barnett J & Carrigy A (1978) Factors affecting patients' responses to hospitalisation. *Journal of Advanced Nursing* **3**: 331.

Wright L (1974) *Bowel Function in Hospital Patients*. London: RCN.

Index